GETTING PREGNANT

Other books in the series
BEING PREGNANT
*by Ruth Steinberg
and Linda Robinson*

the woman's answer book

GETTING PREGNANT

Robert Winston

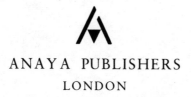

ANAYA PUBLISHERS

LONDON

First published in Great Britain in 1989
by Anaya Publishers Ltd, 49 Neal Street, London WC2H 9PJ

Text Copyright © 1989 Robert Winston
Illustrations Copyright © 1989 Anaya Publishers Ltd

Editor: Nancy Duin
Designer: Susie Home
Illustrator: Sharon Perks

British Library Cataloguing in Publication Data
A CIP catalogue record for this book is available from the British Library.

ISBN 1-85470-002-2

Typeset by Keyspools
Printed and bound in Great Britain by Redwood Burn

Acknowledgements

As always, I owe an immense debt to our patients from whom all of us continue to learn. Their dedication, bravery and singlemindedness commands respect.

I am particularly grateful to Patricia Want, Librarian of the Royal College of Obstetricians and Gynaecologists, who frequently pointed me in the right direction, and to her staff. It was a pleasure to be helped by such an experienced editor as Nancy Duin, and I am conscious of the forbearance of my publishers, Anaya, who were remarkably tolerant when the schedule was tight.

I owe special thanks to my great friend and colleague Mr Raul Margara, without whose solid backing and excellent clinical work I would never have time to publish anything. Last, and most important, my wife Lira has been as loving, supportive and as patient as ever during my prolonged bouts over the keyboard.

Contents

CONTENTS

*To The Lady Young of Graffham,
whose many kindnesses and great
encouragement are deeply
appreciated.*

Introduction

Of all our bodily functions, how we have children is the most remarkable. It is also, in many ways, mysterious. The desire to have children runs deeper than many of us realize or will admit. Whether you are religious or not, it is striking that the first command in the Bible is: "Be fruitful and multiply" (Genesis 1: 28). Why we feel so strongly is not easy to explain.

One thing is clear. By having children, we leave a part of ourselves – our own genetic message which we inherited from our parents and they from their parents – on this planet. Our children are our connection with life that preceded us and that which follows us. It is truly remarkable that the unique collection of genes that we each have, which determine the way we think, the personality we have, the way we look, our abilities and disabilities, are identical to the genes that our ancestors had at the very beginning of human existence. The processes involved in reproduction ensure that the genes of our parents are mixed and randomly assigned to us. These genes are reallocated in successive generations. Nature reshuffles the genetic pack with each conception.

If you think about it, whatever we achieve on this earth – even if we are politicians or Nobel Prize winners – becomes insignificant within 15 years of our death. Try to name six Nobel Prize winners or six leading members of the Government of 15 or 20 years ago – and what they achieved. But no matter how important or insignificant each of us is, we shape the world of the future if we produce a child.

How pregnancy occurs is remarkably complex. In fact, well over half the facts of life are still unknown. Much more research is required before we will know most of what there is to know about getting pregnant. This, above all, is why the treatment of people who have difficulty conceiving a child is so imperfect. My object in writing this book is to try to explain how conception occurs and, if you are having difficulty in conceiving, how to maximize your chances of being one of the lucky 35 per cent. If you are reading this book because you think you may find it difficult to get pregnant, I hope that it will tell you how best to cope with the difficulty.

PART I

Becoming Pregnant

CHAPTER ONE

How a Baby is Conceived

A good way to start learning about conception and how it occurs is to understand the more scientific aspects of human reproduction – how sperm meets egg and how the early embryo implants. Knowledge of this basic biology is fairly essential if we are to make sensible decisions about conception and contraception, and how to maximize the chances of normal development of an early pregnancy. What may come as a surprise is just how big are the gaps in our knowledge.

I have tried three approaches in this chapter. First, I have devoted most space to those parts of human biology which are important medically. For example, to understand what the Fallopian tubes do may seem very unimportant. However, if you are unfortunate in having blocked or damaged tubes, it may help to know what functions and events should be taking place normally.

Second, I have, here and elsewhere, deliberately spent some time discussing animals other than humans. Apart from being interesting in itself, much of the knowledge we have about our own bodies comes from intensive studies of many animal species. Without those, we would be quite unable to make deductions about human physiology or understand how the human body works.

Third, whenever possible I have taken a look at the historical context. The history of our knowledge of human reproduction is extraordinary, fascinating and revealing. It tells us, apart from anything else, that we still suffer from many mistaken ideas even now, in an age of supposed enlightenment and sophistication.

The female reproductive system

The eggs

William Harvey's famous treatise *De generatione animalium (On the reproduction of animals)*, published in 1651, has a delightful frontispiece. The hands of Jove hold an open egg, out of which come forth all forms of life. The egg, which perhaps is the beginning of all life, is as good a point as any for us to start.

Eggs (ova) do not simply grow in a woman's ovaries throughout her reproductive lifetime. The process which produces them begins when the human female embryo is less than 2 millimetres in length – only about 21 days after fertilization. Two millimetres is about half the size of the head of a match. It may seem slightly incredible that anything that small can have an egg in it, but human eggs are very small indeed, about one-tenth of the size of the full stop at the end of this sentence. Nevertheless, they are the largest cells in the human body.

At this stage of development, the female embryo has no clearly identifiable organs, although a primitive heart of some kind could be seen under a microscope. The cells from which the eggs will actually

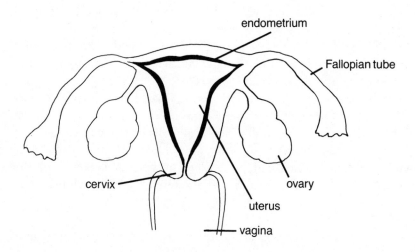

The female reproductive system.

develop are called the *primordial germ cells*. These do not come from the embryo itself, but grow in the structure which in humans is next to the embryo – the *yolk sac*. It is thought that, about three weeks or so after fertilization, these germ cells form up in line and move into the embryo along the structure which later in pregnancy will become the umbilical cord.

This procession of the germ cells is not well understood. Certainly it is very remarkable, for it seems that the germ cells move under their own steam, towards the tissues which will become the ovaries. In studies of animals, using time-lapse photography, the germ cells have been seen to move rather like an amoeba moves. As far as we know, only about 100 germ cells migrate to the area which will become the ovaries, and here they continue to multiply.

The primordial germ cells repeatedly divide, and by the fifth month of life inside the womb, a baby girl has around 7 million eggs in her ovaries. By the time she is born, more than half of these eggs will have died and there will be only about 2 million left, and by puberty, only 200,000–500,000 remain. Of all these, only a few – no more than 400 or 500 (one each month or so) – will actually be ovulated during adult life. During a woman's fertile years – with time off for childbearing and breastfeeding – the maximum number of children she could have is only about 30. According to the *Guinness Book of Records*, the world record is currently held by Mrs McNaught with 22 babies from 22 separate pregnancies. However, in the average adult relationship in the Western world, just two or three eggs will be properly fertilized and become children. When one considers that each of an adult woman's eggs is entirely genetically unique, with different genes derived at random from the woman's mother and father, nature does seem extraordinarily wasteful.

By the time of ovulation, when the egg is shed on its way to be fertilized, it contains only half the normal 46 chromosomes (on which are carried the genes) that all other adult cells have – namely 23. The other 23 will be contributed by the sperm which fertilizes it. These two portions of genes will determine the genetic make-up of the baby, which will decide its unique characteristics as it develops.

The ovaries

The ovaries, where the eggs are stored, were described in 1651 by that great English physician William Harvey, who was very interested in reproduction. He had often accompanied Charles I when the King

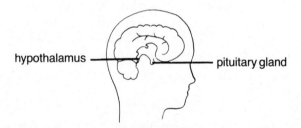

The pituitary gland and the hypothalamus in the brain work together to produce hormones that regulate ovulation.

hunted deer on the royal estates After the deer were killed, Harvey had been able to dissect them. ". . . The female testicles as they are called," he wrote, "whether they be examined before or after intercourse, neither swell nor vary from their usual condition; they show no trace of being of the slightest use either in the business of intercourse or in that of generation." Fellows of the Royal Society, even to this day, get things wrong, and Harvey started a trend. His observations significantly held up progress in the understanding of reproduction. Today, we know much more, despite Harvey. For instance, we know that a girl's ovaries are hardly active at all during childhood. The length of time that the eggs remain in the ovaries in humans may be of particular significance. We know that both the primordial germ cells and the early eggs are very sensitive to certain physical stimuli – such as radiation. The fact that, in humans, the eggs shed towards the end of reproductive life will have been in the ovary for 40 years or longer may have some bearing on why older women are at greater risk of conceiving a genetically damaged child.

The ovaries remain immature and relatively inactive until puberty, when the pituitary gland – the "master" of all the hormone-producing endocrine glands – starts to send messages to them. The pituitary gland, which is about the size of a small bean, is under the brain about an inch (3 cm) behind the eye sockets. Precisely what tells the pituitary gland to start sending hormone messages is not fully understood. It seems that the hypothalamus, a control centre in the brain about 3 inches (7.5 cm) behind the pituitary, plays a crucial role. The hormones which the pituitary produces are *follicle-stimulating hormone* (FSH) and *luteinizing hormone* (LH).

Follicle-stimulating hormone is responsible for stimulating eggs to become· mature. I pointed out earlier that there will be many thousands of eggs in each ovary. All of these inactive eggs are exposed to FSH from the pituitary at the time of puberty, but we do not understand why only a few of them start to respond to the stimulus to develop. Each egg which matures does so inside a small blister-like structure – the *Graafian follicle* – which is filled with fluid. The egg usually grows to one side of the follicle, where it is surrounded by helper cells – the *granulosa cells*.

Most eggs remain inactive and never develop inside an expanding follicle. Only those that do are capable of ovulation – that is, capable of leaving one of the ovaries and travelling through a Fallopian tube to be fertilized by a sperm. Each month, about 20 eggs, each within a follicle, start to mature, but in humans only one follicle becomes "dominant" and goes on to become fully mature and to ovulate. As far as we know, the dominant follicle controls the growth of the other follicles and prevents them from getting large enough to ovulate. Consequently, they actually shrink and the egg inside them dies. Only a few other mammals make a single dominant follicle; most produce several eggs at one ovulation. This is why cats and rabbits, for example, produce litters.

The granulosa cells, which surround each egg and line each follicle, perform two functions. First, they are responsible for feeding the egg with nutrients. The egg is virtually a perfect sphere with quite a smooth surface, and therefore it has the smallest surface area possible for its size. Yet it is highly active and consumes a lot of energy – especially when finally maturing, just before ovulation. On the face of it, it might seem as if God didn't do a particularly good job in designing the egg because it has little to call on within its own structure to provide the energy it needs. However, the 7 million or more granulosa cells which are packed into each follicle are there partly to look after each egg. Their total surface area increases hugely the amount of energy which is available to the egg by absorption. This remarkable phenomenon must be the only example in the body of one virtually invisible cell being serviced by many millions of others.

The second major function of the granulosa cells is to manufacture oestrogen. Oestrogen is the female hormone which stimulates breast development, female body shape and fat, and the other female secondary sex characteristics. As we shall see later, the levels of oestrogen in the body rise and fall during the menstrual cycle, depending on the number and activity of the granulosa cells.

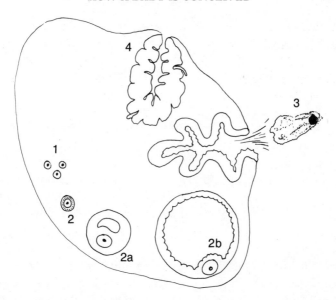

The development of a follicle containing the egg. (1) Immature eggs. (2, 2a & 2b) Maturing Graafian follicle and egg. (3) Rupture of follicle with release of egg surrounded by granulosa cells (ovulation). (4) Corpus luteum about 4-5 days after ovulation.

Ovulation

Ovulation is the process during which the egg leaves the ovary – in humans, roughly halfway between two menstrual periods. In all mammals, this process is controlled by the hormones from the pituitary gland: LH and FSH. As we have seen, FSH stimulates the follicle to grow to its maximum, before ovulation. LH then stimulates the follicle to open and release the egg. How does the body know when to send the LH signal? There is a wonderful mechanism here. Understanding this helps us to understand what goes wrong when women fail to ovulate.

As FSH stimulates the follicle to grow, the granulosa cells (which produce oestrogen) increase in number and activity. As the granulosa cells increase, so does the manufacture of oestrogen. Eventually oestrogen output is high and some of it gets into the bloodstream. This rise in oestrogen in the blood stimulates the brain, telling the hypothalamus that the follicle is now mature and ready to release a ripe egg. An immediate message is then sent from the hypothalamus to the pituitary gland. The pituitary responds by sending out a sharp pulse of LH, and approximately 36 hours after the rise of LH in the blood, ovulation occurs. This process – that is, the rise of one hormone prompting the secretion of another and so on – is called a "feedback" mechanism.

Immature eggs will not normally fertilize. If they do, fertilization produces an abnormal embryo which cannot survive or implant in the womb (uterus) properly. One of the functions of the feedback mechanism is to ensure that, as far as possible, only a ripe egg leaves the ovary at ovulation. The mature egg has chromosomes at the right stage for further development. It also is capable of taking in a single sperm and blocking the entry of all other sperm which may be surrounding it. In addition, a mature egg is able to process the head of the sperm which enters it, to ensure that the egg and sperm subsequently fuse successfully. An understanding of these principles is essential to an understanding of human fertility and the treatment of infertility. The need for a mature egg explains why drugs given to encourage ovulation must be given in the right sequence and with the right timing. Without this, abnormal embryos are likely to be produced, which are not able to form a pregnancy.

The egg after ovulation

Once the egg has left its follicle, it hopefully will find its way into one of the two Fallopian tubes. The end of each tube lies very close to the surface of one of the ovaries. Whether or not the tube actively picks up the egg is unknown. It probably does, as the lining of the tube is covered with very fine hair-like structures – *cilia* – which beat rhythmically, wafting any nearby particles into the tube itself. These cilia seem to be quite important as they undoubtedly provide one of the ways in which eggs are transported down the tube and eventually into the uterus. When the cilia are damaged or missing – for example, after a tubal infection – a woman may be infertile or prone to ectopic pregnancy (*see* Chapter 13).

The egg has other assistance in its journey to meet the sperm. Immediately after ovulation, the egg is surrounded by some of the granulosa cells from the ovary. These cells, which resemble a sunburst, probably help the egg find its way into the tube because they are very sticky and adhere to the tubal surface. Once the egg is in the tube, it is ready to meet the sperm.

People frequently wonder what happens if the egg does not, or cannot, find its way into the tube. This may be the situation, for example, if the tubes are blocked. In practice, it is very likely that eggs are frequently lost outside the tube. Even though they are the biggest single cells in the body, they are still very tiny – invisible to the naked eye – and they simply get lost within the abdomen, where they disintegrate.

Let us now leave the egg, hopefully in the Fallopian tube, and return to the ovary.

The ovary after ovulation

Following ovulation, the follicle from which the egg came tends to fill with blood. This is one of the reasons why women sometimes feel some pain at the time of ovulation, although, to be fair, this pain can occasionally occur before ovulation. This blood forms a clot and is replaced with fibre-like tissue. The remaining granulosa cells, in addition to producing oestrogen, now start to produce a second hormone, *progesterone*. The production of progesterone is stimulated by the release of LH from the pituitary gland which occurred immediately before ovulation. As we shall see later, progesterone is the hormone which prepares the uterus for implantation of the developing embryo, if fertilization occurs successfully.

The granulosa cells also make an orange-yellow pigment. This is quite vivid in colour, and it stains the entire ruptured follicle. The resulting structure is called a *corpus luteum* (literally "yellow body" in Latin). This yellow appearance was first noted in 1562 by the great Italian anatomist Gabriele Fallopius (who was the first to describe the tubes that were then named after him), but it wasn't until 1697 that the name *corpus luteum* was coined, by another famous anatomist, Marcello Malpighi, after he had described its detailed appearance in the cow. Its function has only recently been understood, and today research still goes on about precisely what it does. The *corpus luteum* is certainly a most important structure, as not only does it produce the progesterone needed to prepare the uterus for a possible pregnancy, but its progesterone production is essential for the earliest development of any embryo which forms. If the corpus luteum is damaged, an early pregnancy may miscarry.

Menstruation

Why is it that human females menstruate, unlike the so-called "lower" animals? All female mammals need to prepare the uterus so

21

that a pregnancy will implant. In lower animals, there is an *oestrus cycle* – where the female comes on to heat and is receptive to the male. During this phase, which may be very frequent or very infrequent – once every four days in guinea pigs, once a year in hippopotamuses – the lining of the uterus is prepared for the possible reception of a pregnancy.

In the evolution of humans and certain others of the monkey family, the oestrus cycle has been replaced by the menstrual cycle. Perhaps because, in humans, sexual intercourse is usually much more of a cerebral process (and not just a question of rutting), women do not simply become physically receptive to men as females of other species do to males. In humans, the female has far more control. It is the development of this degree of control which seems to have led to the evolution of the menstrual cycle.

Until the 19th century, it was often supposed that women usually ovulated at the time of menstruation. This idea was based on the evidence that women who did not menstruate were usually infertile. It was also recognized that animals, who went through an oestrus period, ovulated at this time.

A clue to the truth was found in the post-mortem room. Although it was generally agreed that ovulation occurred during menstruation, doctors and scientists were puzzled because, during autopsies of women who had been menstruating at the time of their deaths, they could find little sign of any ovarian activity – and it was known that the egg developed in a follicle, a structure very obvious to the naked eye. On the other hand, follicles were sometimes seen at post-mortem in women who had not had a menstrual period for several years. In spite of these essentially conflicting pieces of evidence, doctors remained convinced that ovulation coincided with menstruation. Dr Pouchet, writing in Paris in 1842, stated that "in the intermenstrual phase ... conception is physically impossible."

This led Dr Raciborski, also of Paris, to an ingenious idea. He interrogated a group of young women, all who had (presumably) been virgins before their marriages and who became pregnant within two months of their weddings. The majority of those marrying within a few days of the end of their period conceived immediately. Those who married 10–18 days after a period never conceived until the following month. Thus Dr Raciborski arrived successfully at the correct time of human ovulation. It says something for the stubborn nature of the medical profession that his observations were largely

22

ignored. It is also interesting to think that, with the changes in sexual morality and the availability of contraception, his observations could not have been made in our present society.

Why you do not menstruate during pregnancy

The *corpus luteum* breaks down (degenerates) if it receives no stimulus. As LH production from the pituitary gland falls after ovulation, there is no longer any stimulus to the ovary, so the *corpus luteum* withers and progesterone production falls. The fall in progesterone leads to a loss of stimulus to the uterus, and its blood-filled lining therefore also withers. This produces menstrual bleeding. If a pregnancy occurs, the embryo produces the hormone *human chorionic gonadotrophin* (HCG). HCG is almost identical in chemical structure to LH, so similar, in fact, that the *corpus luteum* cannot tell the difference. Consequently, in the event of pregnancy, the *corpus luteum* is maintained, progesterone output carries on, the lining of the uterus continues to be stimulated and menstruation does not occur.

The male reproductive system

The production of sperm

Unlike eggs, which are present in the ovaries from before birth, spermatozoa, or sperm, are first manufactured at puberty. They are made in the two testes (or testicles), the organs which hang inside the scrotum. The testes are filled with thousands of microscopic little tubes, inside which the sperm grow (*see below*). These minute tubes are connected to yet more tubes, called the *rete testis*. *Rete* is Latin for "a net", and this term was given to this structure presumably because the fine tubes form a network in the testes. The tubes in the rete testis are thought to produce special fluids, important for sperm development. The rete in each testicle is connected to yet more tubes, called the *efferent ducts*, of which there are about eight. These efferent ducts lead into one single tube, the *epididymis*, which is itself a pretty amazing bit of plumbing.

The epididymis is a remarkably coiled tube, approximately 40 feet (12 m) in length. It has an extremely fine inner diameter, or bore, being thinner in total width than a fine piece of thread. Sperm are transported along this tubing, which is their only way to the outside world. At the beginning of their journey, they cannot move on their own; the epididymis itself is responsible for their transport by means of gentle muscular contractions in its wall. However, the epididymis does not simply transport the sperm; it also modifies them. During their travels through the epididymis, which takes two to three weeks, the sperm become capable of fertilization, and some ill-understood process takes place whereby the sperm gain the ability to move (*motility*). By the end of their journey, they are able to swim under their own power.

The epididymis, then, is a complex and essential reproductive organ. If it is damaged, sperm may not be able to develop normally and may be incapable of fertilization. If blocked – even in only one tiny place – all sperm production from that testicle is useless.

The epididymis is joined to yet another tube, the *vas deferens*. This is a thicker, more muscular tube about $\frac{1}{6}$ inch (4 mm) thick. The vas deferens is the final piece of tubing by which the sperm leave the scrotum. It can just be felt in most men by rolling it gently between finger and thumb in the groin, where the scrotum joins the abdominal skin.

Why do the testicles hang outside a man's body?

In many mammals, but by no means all, the testicles descend from the abdominal cavity into a scrotum during early childhood. Once outside, they are considerably cooler than they would be inside. The temperature in the scrotum is usually as much as 8.5–15°F (4–7°C) below the general body temperature. Moreover, the blood vessels to the testicles are coiled in a highly complex way, so that by the time the blood arrives in the scrotum, it is much cooler than normal.

It is widely thought that the cooler temperature of the scrotum is essential for sperm production. It is this idea which leads to many men, with poor sperm counts, being asked to take regular cold baths. This advice is of dubious value as there is little evidence that testicular cooling will do any good – after all, no man can sit in a cold bath all day! If you have been given this advice and you are reluctant to use cold water on this sensitive region, think of the bull elephant whose testicles are completely inside the abdomen, not, I think, to the detriment of his power of procreation.

The final stage of the journey

Unlike the epididymis in the scrotum, the vas deferens moves the

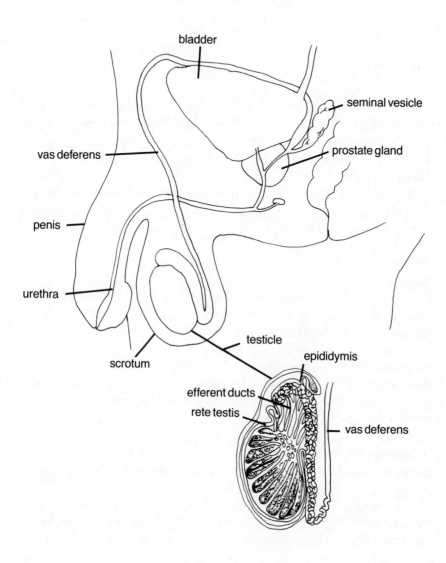

The male reproductive system.

sperm along quite rapidly. It contracts during male orgasm and transports sperm past the *seminal vesicles* and the *prostate gland* into the urethra. The urethra is the tube which connects the bladder to the outside world, through the penis. During ejaculation, the connection between the urethra and the bladder is shut off, and semen containing sperm is rapidly transported along it.

The semen

The semen is at first partly fluid, partly solid. It contains the sperm and a fluid component from the seminal vesicles and from the prostate gland. Some fluid is also contributed by glands in the urethra itself. All this fluid is essential to provide the sperm with energy. Men who have a damaged prostate or damaged seminal vesicles may be infertile. The solid component containing the sperm is in the form of a jelly and after ejaculation it remains in this form for up to 30 minutes. Liquefaction (the "melting" of this jelly caused by a special chemical process) is necessary before the sperm are capable of release into the female genital tract.

Ejaculation

During orgasm, ejaculation follows a vigorous pumping action of the muscles at the base of the penis. In certain rare cases of infertility, these muscles may not work properly. The total volume of semen – the *ejaculate* – should usually be about 1–8 millilitres (an average teaspoon holds about 5 millilitres of fluid). If there is too little fluid, the man may be infertile because there is not enough fluid to get the sperm into the female system; too much and the sperm may be too diluted. However, on the whole, the precise volume is usually not all that important, and is nothing for you and your partner to get worried about – certainly there is no need to raid the kitchen drawer for measuring spoons. Interestingly, most of the sperm are contained in the first part of ejaculation; the rest is just surplus fluid.

In some animals, such as rodents, the ejaculate remains solid for a considerable length of time, forming a jelly plug that fills the the female's vagina. The quantity of fluid ejaculated varies considerably from species to species: in mice, only a minute droplet is ejaculated, while pigs may produce a cupful. The length of sexual intercourse also varies hugely: in bulls and rabbits it is over in a matter of seconds, while camels take 24 hours, which must be a source of great satisfaction in arid and featureless deserts.

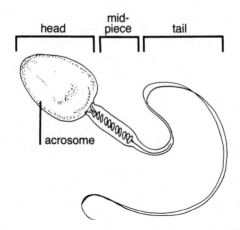

The sperm

Just as the egg is the largest cell in the body, the sperm are the smallest. They were first described in 1678 by Anthony van Leeuwenhoek, when he examined semen (possibly his own) using a primitive microscope of his own design and making. Actually, as frequently happens in science, Van Leeuwenhoek, although credited with the discovery of human sperm, was not actually the first to see them. Nowadays it is largely forgotten that probably the first person to see sperm was Dr Louis de Ham in 1667, who had been using a microscope to study the nocturnal emissions of a patient with gonorrhoea. He then told Van Leeuwenhoek of his discovery of moving spermatozoa. The latter published a full description of his own findings, calling the sperm "animalcules". It rapidly became fashionable in well-to-do society for men to examine their own semen, and soon many people believed they could see a fully formed human figure (a *homunculus*) in the head of the sperm. Some people even wrote of having discovered male and female sperm under the microscope; others imagined they could see the sperm intertwined in microscopic intercourse or even pregnant.

It was really only with the modern invention of the electron microscope that really detailed information about sperm was acquired. A sperm comprises three major parts and may be thought of as rather like a missile:

• *the head* is equivalent to a missile's warhead and contains the sperm's genetic message. Just like the unfertilized egg, this consists of 23 chromosomes – half the number needed for normal cells. The head is surrounded by a cap, the *acrosome*, which is not removed

27

until after the sperm is capacitated (*see below*) and ready to fertilize the egg. Removal of this cap is rather like the arming of a warhead.

• *the mid-piece* is very complex in structure and may be likened to the sperm's fuel storage and the computer systems that control its movements.

• *the tail*, which moves like a whiplash, provides the propulsive force which moves the sperm forward. The force of this whiplash increases greatly when the sperm is close to its target, the egg, when the sperm accelerates considerably.

How egg and sperm meet

During sexual intercourse, the average man ejaculates between 100 million and 300 million sperm into the vagina. Quite remarkably, just as each human egg is unique, each of these sperm is genetically unique. Each contains a different set of genes, derived from those of the man, and, depending upon which sperm finally hits which egg, the resulting baby will exhibit its unique, individual characteristics.

This number of sperm may seem enormous, especially when you realize that only one is required to fertilize an egg. Some species, such as pigs and cattle, actually produce far more – several thousand million at a single ejaculation. Many sperm are required because of the perilous journey they now undertake. How the egg and sperm finally meet is by no means simple.

To start with, many sperm simply fall out of the vagina. This is quite natural, but it can be of great concern to infertile couples who imagine that something abnormal is happening to them.

Then, the vagina itself is relatively hostile to sperm. The vaginal secretions are rather acid, an environment in which sperm usually do not survive. It may seem strange that nature has allowed the vagina to be acid, as reception of sperm is obviously crucial for the survival of the species. But this acidity also protects against bacteria and dangerous infection, and thus prevents damage to the lining of the womb and tubes.

Some sperm – perhaps no more than 5 per cent – find their way into the mucus that covers the neck of the womb, or *cervix*. This mucus tends to be thin, watery and penetrable to sperm near the time of ovulation. Here, two important things happen to the sperm. First, they are protected, not only against the acids in the vagina, but also against the woman's white blood cells, including the *phagocytes*. These scavenging cells, which normally protect the body against invasion by bacteria and other foreign material, are not usually active in healthy cervical mucus around the time of ovulation. Second, during physical contact with the mucus, each sperm undergoes a quite mysterious process called *capacitation*, in which the sperm cap (the acrosome) is removed. Only when this has happened is the sperm capable of penetrating an egg. Within five to ten minutes of ejaculation, some sperm pass through the cervical mucus, through the uterus, and into the tubes, where they are ready to fertilize an egg. The remaining sperm in the cervical pool of mucus stay there for many hours – certainly 72 hours and possibly much longer – with sperm constantly being passed up into the uterus and then the tubes.

However, few sperm get into the uterus. Just how few is uncertain. We know that, in rabbits, perhaps not more than 0.5 per cent make it through the cervix. The situation is likely to be quite similar in women. Therefore, of the 300 million that arrive in the vagina, no more than 1–2 million at most get as far as the uterus.

The uterus is also a hostile environment. Here there are many phagocytes, protective against infection, which recognize the sperm as foreign invaders and thus set out to destroy them. Only a small fraction of sperm get into the Fallopian tube. At any one time, after intercourse, probably no more than about 200 sperm will be present.

Passage of sperm into the Fallopian tube seems a complicated affair. They do not just swim there. They are actively transported, probably by muscular contractions of the uterus and tubes. We know this because the speed at which human sperm swim has been carefully measured. Considering the tiny size of the sperm, the distance from the cervix to the tube is huge and if sperm were left to their own travel arrangements, they would not arrive in the tube until seven or more hours after intercourse. In fact, sperm get into the tube within five minutes after being deposited in the vagina; this has been demonstrated in volunteers undergoing surgery on their Fallopian tubes. It is interesting to consider that, while the tube is transporting sperm in one direction – towards the ovary – it is simultaneously transporting the egg in precisely the opposite direction – towards the uterus and therefore the sperm pool. A complex tube, indeed.

As well as transporting sperm, the Fallopian tube also acts as a filter. The human male is an unusual animal in that he tends to produce many abnormal sperm in his ejaculate. The first part of the tube – the *isthmus* – appears to trap dead and abnormal sperm so that only normal ones arrive in the upper part – the *ampulla*.

Because sperm can live for quite long periods both in the cervical mucus and in the tubal fluids means that careful timing of intercourse just before ovulation is almost certainly unnecessary. It is important to understand this, because recognition of this fact takes some of the sting out of being infertile. Many couples trying to conceive get very worried about timing intercourse. This makes sexual intercourse a far cry from love-making and creates a great strain for some people. Just how long the sperm are capable of fertilizing an egg after intercourse is unknown – perhaps two days or so. We know for certain that, in some species, sperm retain their viability for long periods. In some bats, for instance, sperm are definitely known to be retained in the uterus for several months after intercourse and are still able to cause a pregnancy. In a particular strain of mouse, the female can become pregnant with two successive litters after a single act of insemination. This is evidence that some of the sperm survive in the glands of the uterus throughout pregnancy before being finally allowed to fertilize eggs.

Fertilization and development of the embryo

Fertilization – the stages during which the sperm enters the egg and fuses with it and the egg starts dividing – takes place in the Fallopian tube. Fertilization is not a single instantaneous process: in humans, it takes place over the best part of 24 hours. For entirely healthy fertilization to occur, the egg has to be properly mature. If it is "under-ripe", a sperm may not enter it properly; if "over-ripe", more than one sperm may enter it, causing an abnormal number of chromosomes (i.e. more than 46), which is incompatible with life.

A mature egg has its chromosomes ready for cell division, and its chemistry ready to utilize the energy needed for subsequent cell division. A mature egg is also capable of only allowing a single sperm to penetrate it: remarkably, as soon as one sperm has penetrated, a normally mature egg throws up a chemical barrier which prevents other sperm from entering it. An abnormal or immature egg may divide into what may seem to be a normal embryo, but the embryo so formed will not go on to become a live baby. The factors which decide whether an egg is mature or not are largely hormonal; it is for this reason that measurement of a woman's hormones during "test-tube baby" (*in vitro* fertilization, IVF) treatment is so important.

30

Those IVF programmes in which blood hormone levels are not measured regularly (all too common, I'm afraid) may be unable to detect when the eggs that have been stimulated are properly mature (*see* Chapter 10).

I stressed earlier that fertilization is not an immediate process, but takes place over very many hours in a series of stages. This is important, not only biologically but also, I think, morally. Those who maintain that human life begins at conception or, more precisely, fertilization, and that the resulting embryo is in some way sacrosanct – while the egg is not – may pause to consider. If life begins at the moment of fertilization, precisely which moment is considered the important one?

The fertilized egg develops in the tube. During the first 24 hours, it divides once into two cells. During the next day, each of those cells divides. Each cell division occurs at intervals of about 15 hours so that, by the end of two days there are four to eight cells, and by the time 90 hours have elapsed there are usually somewhere around 64 cells. In the early stages of human development – that is, when the embryo comprises up to about eight cells – each cell has what is known as *totipotential*. This simply means that each cell contains all the capability of developing into a human being. Thus, if the eight-cell embryo was deliberately divided into its eight independent cells, which were then left to grow separately, potentially eight human beings – each, incidentally, identical – could develop. This is the mechanism by which identical twins occur: occasionally, the embryo divides completely into two, quite spontaneously.

The ability of each early embryonic cell to develop into a person is of considerable importance to women undergoing IVF treatment. Quite commonly, an embryo with several of its total number of cells fragmented or dying may be put deliberately into the uterus. Occasionally, seven cells out of a total of eight may show signs of not being viable. This does not necessarily prevent a perfectly normal pregnancy occurring, provided the one remaining cell is quite healthy. Another interesting fact is that an embryo, when it arrives in the uterus 96 hours or so after fertilization, is composed of approximately 64–100 cells. Most of these cells, perhaps 85 per cent of them, become the membranes (in which the baby lives) and placenta (which nourishes it), and these are thrown away at birth! Only a very few cells, those comprising the so-called *inner cell mass*, actually develop into the embryo proper.

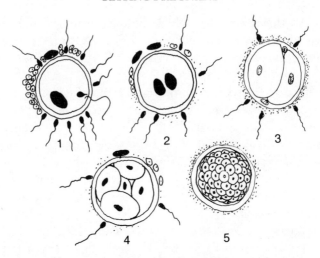

Fertilization and early embryonic development. (1) Just one sperm enters the egg and others are immediately "locked out". The tail of the fertilizing sperm breaks off. (2) Two pronuclei form about 15 hours after sperm entry and are only visible for a few hours. (3) The first division of the egg into two cells is completed in about 24-40 hours. (4) By two to three days the embryo may be approximately eight cells, each potentially capable of developing into a person. (5) By about 80 hours the blastocyst is formed, containing perhaps 50-100 cells.

It is worth pointing out that an egg may divide into separate cells without ever having been exposed to a sperm. If this happens, the egg looks to all intents and purposes like a perfectly normal embryo. This independent cell division, or *cleavage*, may be stimulated by exposure to electric shock, sudden changes in temperature or alteration in the chemical environment surrounding the egg; it can also happen without any obvious stimulus. Such cleaving eggs, at least in mammals, are not capable of development beyond a certain stage. For one thing, most of them will not have the correct number of chromosomes. However, in frogs, such a cleaved egg (which has never even seen a sperm) is capable of developing into a perfectly healthy adult frog – a true example of virgin birth. Spontaneous cleavage of eggs is important because an unfertilized but cleaved egg may be mistakenly transferred to the uterus during test-tube baby treatment. Unless the egg is examined approximately 18 hours after exposure to sperm, it is not possible to know until later whether an egg (which may appear to have become a normal embryo) has really been fertilized. For this reason, the best test-tube baby clinics always examine all eggs about

32

18 hours after insemination, to ensure that only potentially viable embryos will later be transferred.

After the human embryo enters the uterus, it floats around for approximately two or three days. Up until this stage, although its cells have been constantly dividing and multiplying, it will not have grown physically in size at all. It is still the same size as the original egg cell because each cell which has been formed has been smaller than the last. It is now a clump or ball of cells, with a central cavity filled with fluid. The technical name for this stage of development is a *blastocyst*. The embryo only starts to increase in size around six or seven days after fertilization, just about the time when it starts to stick to the lining of the uterus, the *endometrium*.

Not all mammals follow the same pattern as humans. In some species, the free-floating embryo at the blastocyst stage goes into a kind of suspended animation – so-called "diapause". This period of suspension of all growth or activity varies considerably from species to species: in roe deer, the embryo almost stops all development for five months and pregnancy lasts for a total of about ten months. In European badgers, the embryo halts all growth at this stage for ten months, being simply retained in the mother's uterus. The longest example of suspended animation is in the wallaby, a member of the kangaroo family, where embryonic growth is halted for up to a year. Why diapause should occur in some species is not entirely known, but it is widely believed that this is an adaptation to a harsh environment, and prevents young being born during the depths of a bitter winter, when their chances of survival would be seriously limited.

Implantation of the embryo

At seven days after fertilization, the human embryo starts to implant into the endometrium. Precisely how this happens is not at all well understood at present. It is a major area of research, one that has the most important implications in our understanding of normal fertility, infertility, miscarriage and contraception, and one in which we can, hopefully, expect greater progress during the next decade. The embryo appears to control its own implantation, and, apparently it does this by secreting the pregnancy hormone *human chorionic gonadotrophin* (HCG). As we have already seen, this is the hormone which is very similar in structure to the pituitary hormone LH, which stimulates the ovary to make progesterone.

HCG appears to influence the lining of the uterus to receive the

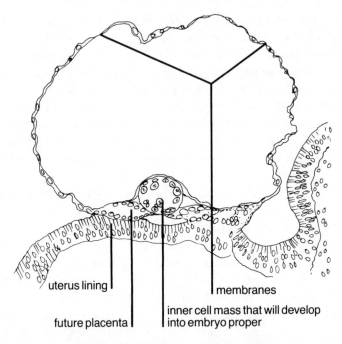

uterus lining

membranes

future placenta

inner cell mass that will develop into embryo proper

The start of implantation of a 7-day embryo into the lining of the uterus, here seen in cross-section magnified 600 times. Most of the embryonic cells form the placenta and membranes, and only about one-tenth will become a person (if implantation succeeds).

embryo and allow it to implant. HCG can be detected soon after this stage by very sensitive pregnancy tests on blood – even before the next menstrual period is due. Implantation is a very remarkable event. If you think about it, the embryo is completely foreign. It is going to become an individual quite different from its mother, with its own blood group, tissue type and special proteins. However, it is not rejected by the mother's body. It is, in fact, the perfect transplant – the perfect parasite. No other foreign material is ever accepted as readily, because the body's natural defence mechanisms will prevent it. This extraordinary phenomenon is very poorly understood.

Early embryonic development and implantation are very precarious. We know that at least 40 per cent of human embryos simply do not make it beyond this stage, but why this is so is not clear. Moreover, many other embryos are lost at the time of menstruation, just as early implantation is completed; this, too, is not understood.

If a woman has a slightly delayed, heavier-than-usual period, this may signify that a very early pregnancy has been lost. If you occasionally experience delayed cycles when you think you have definitely ovulated, you may well be getting pregnant, but losing the early embryo. It is well worth finding out if you are actually conceiving. A sensitive blood test for HCG may reassure you that you are at least capable of getting pregnant – especially after tubal surgery, for example, when this knowledge will give you real and genuine hope.

By 14 days, the tiny embryo is firmly implanted in the uterine lining. Although miscarriage can still happen, it is now much less likely, and it becomes progressively less common the further a pregnancy develops (*see* Chapter 13). It is at this point that the organs of the embryo first start to develop. The "primitive streak", the beginning of the nervous system, is the first identifiable structure. The heart starts to form at around 23 days and other organs follow. The baby has a clearly defined human shape by about ten weeks, when it is almost 1 inch (2.5 cm) long and weighs about $\frac{1}{4}$ ounce (7 g).

CHAPTER TWO

Timing Your Pregnancy

Few people consciously plan a pregnancy, and children are seldom worse off for that. I am not at all sure that firmly planning when to start a family really makes much sense for most people. Apart from any other consideration, the vagaries of our biology and the fact that humans are the most naturally infertile of all mammals makes the achievement of a pregnancy an imprecise and unpredictable event.

Whenever you do have your first baby, life will become different in a way you cannot completely imagine and certainly will not anticipate. Looking after a new person gives you extraordinary responsibilities and is, apart from anything else, a most maturing influence. These responsibilities are not that easy to predict, and therefore nobody can plan so perfectly that they will be able to cope with all the changes in their lives. Having a baby changes how you think about yourself, as well as your partner. It may alter your relationship with your own parents, change your views about some friendships and will almost certainly (at least temporarily) change your interests in life, focus your ambitions and alter your attitude to your job. No matter how consciously you take the decision to have a baby, this time of major change in your life is not something which you can plan completely.

Making your decision

Most couples will want to discuss having a baby well before the event. Some books advise you to work out how starting a family will change your lives, and some couples even map out how they will divide responsibility for the baby. However, to my mind, this does not make much sense before pregnancy. Inevitably, a special bond between mother and baby develops. A mother's closeness to her child after birth and the act of breast-feeding are both facts of life that inevitably exclude the man to some extent. Following the birth of a child, men will take on a role that cannot be entirely predicted.

I am reasonably certain about at least one thing. Getting pregnant is generally a poor way of cementing a failing relationship. Of the unhappy infertile women who come to me, desperate to have treatment to get pregnant, many tell me that they are terrified that their relationship with their partner cannot survive unless they have a baby. It is sad to see how often women believe that, by having a baby, they will prevent their partners leaving them. In my experience, having a baby doesn't help. I have seen people go through endless treatments to get pregnant – surgery and test-tube baby treatment included – but the final success often heralds the beginning of the break-up of their relationship.

Happiness is not ensured by having children. Children can be wonderful but they also disrupt your life, are often noisy, frequently messy, involve extra work and cost money. They also usually reduce a woman's opportunities for independence outside the home and interrupt many promising careers. Certainly, one aspect that you and your partner may need to discuss is that of money. You may have to reckon with a reduced income, and it is a sensible idea to plan your finances before getting pregnant.

Leaving it until later

Some women put off having a baby because they are developing a career. If you are in a fulfilling or exacting job, having a baby can be a great intrusion. If you are just getting established, having a baby may interrupt your chance of success. In addition, many women find it very difficult to get back to full-time work after having children. For all these reasons, most obstetricians have the impression that, more than ever before, they are looking after more women in their late 30s or even early 40s, who are having their first babies.

Other women may conceive later in childbearing life for quite different reasons. An older woman may not be able to get satisfying work that is equal to her enthusiasm or abilities. Some people in this situation choose to get pregnant as a kind of consolation, but this may be a short-term solution to the problem, once the child starts going to school. I also meet many couples who delay having a child till later on in life because one or the other had an unhappy childhood. A feeling of not wishing to perpetuate a bad experience makes many women and men reluctant to commence a family until very late.

Another reason for starting pregnancy at a later age may be that you simply cannot imagine the future without children. This can be a remarkably sudden feeling which people, women especially, experience in their later 30s. This may happen after years of feeling quite remote from any idea of a pregnancy, particularly if you are contemplating life with a new partner.

Mary, a determined and talented journalist, decided at 28 that she never wanted children. Her feeling of certainty was absolute, and her husband also had no desire to have children. To Mary the very idea of pregnancy was off-putting, but most contraceptive methods caused her unpleasant side-effects. Eventually she decided on sterilization – but because she was still so relatively young, she could find no gynaecologist prepared to go along with the idea. Convinced that what she did with her own body was her affair and after reading an advertisement in a newspaper, she turned up at a private family planning agency and requested sterilization. After a five-minute consultation, she entered a private clinic for an overnight stay. Clips were placed across both of her Fallopian tubes in a 15-minute operation, fortunately a relatively reversible procedure.

Thirteen years later, when Mary was 41 and divorced, she fell in love with another man. She felt that she would be failing him totally if she could not offer him children. She could not bring herself to tell him that her tubes had been clipped. Although strongly advised to tell him the truth beforehand, she went through a major operation to have the sterilization reversed without his being informed about why the surgery was being done. She gave all the nurses in the hospital strict instructions not to let the cat out of the bag. So far, sadly, she has not conceived.

In Chapter 5, we will look at some of the physical implications of embarking on pregnancy later in life.

Controlling your fertility

You may be worried that your method of contraception might make it difficult to conceive after stopping. Is there any evidence for this?

The oral contraceptive pill

"The pill" is frequently blamed for making people infertile. However, studies by the Royal College of General Practitioners in Britain show that 80 per cent of all women who have never had a baby, and 90 per cent of those that have, will have conceived within one year of stopping the pill. This is exactly the same proportion of pregnancies found in those who have not used contraception previously. Nor does the length of time you have been on the pill matter.

Some women (about 1 per cent) do stop having periods after coming off the pill, and consequently they have difficulty conceiving afterwards, but this percentage is exactly the same as you would expect to find in an equivalent population not taking the pill. However, just to be safe, most doctors would agree that, if you have very infrequent periods, you may be better off not using the pill.

Starting a pregnancy after stopping the pill

Once you stop the pill, you may ovulate immediately. Alternatively, you may go several weeks before your normal menstrual cycle restarts. If you are one of the rare 1 per cent whose periods do not return within three months, you should visit your family doctor. Treatment is usually very simple, requiring a "fertility pill" (*see* p. 136). A few women may need stronger drugs, given by injection, to stimulate their ovaries more vigorously (*see* pp. 138–41).

Some women, on the other hand, appear to become more fertile on stopping the pill. This so-called "rebound fertility" is somewhat disputed, but there does seem to be limited evidence for it. Certainly, in our laboratories, when rats were given the hormones contained in the pill – which were then stopped abruptly – they were more than normally fertile immediately afterwards, tending to have more babies in a litter. This effect was only temporary.

Because the pill tends to have a somewhat unpredictable effect on ovulation, most obstetricians think it wise for women to avoid getting pregnant immediately after stopping oral contraception. Many doctors advise that you wait until you have had at least two periods before trying to conceive, if only because it makes accurate dating of the pregnancy easier. However, now that we have very precise ways of measuring the early progress of pregnancy with ultrasound (*see* p. 225), I personally think that this really doesn't matter.

One further point. Some recent reports have suggested that a miscarriage is a bit more likely in women who conceive immediately on stopping oral contraceptives. The evidence for this is, to my mind, unconvincing. Miscarriage is an extremely common event and it is probable that the group of women who participated in these studies were monitored so closely that early miscarriages, which normally might well have gone unnoticed (at least by a doctor), were recorded and presumed to be an effect of the pill.

Injectable hormones

Some publicity has been given recently to trials of contraceptive hormones given by injection. The hormones involved are mostly a form of synthetic progesterone (such as Depo-Provera) and are used by comparatively few women. The advantages of this method of contraception are the relative safety of these injections and the fact that one injection will last for several months – very satisfactory if you tend to be the forgetful sort. This kind of drug has not found wide acceptance because, in spite of its undoubted safety, there is some risk of weight gain and irregular bleeding, and because quite a few women only return to normal fertility several months after ceasing the injections. These hormones are therefore not very suitable if you feel you might want to get pregnant at a particular time.

The intrauterine device (IUD) – the "coil"

There is no particular reason why you should not try to become pregnant as soon as you have had an IUD, or coil, removed. However, it may be unwise to use the coil if you have never been pregnant. In recent years, however, there has been something of a question mark over fertility after coil removal. In general, fertility does not seem to be impaired after removal – a large study in the United States in 1968 showed that 60 per cent of women conceived within three months, and that 85 per cent had conceived within a year. These figures were also borne out by a study by the World Health Organization, which looked at women from many different countries; the percentage of women getting pregnant was about that expected in a normal population.

Timing a pregnancy

You may think that people have only recently become interested in controlling family size and in timing pregnancy. On the contrary,

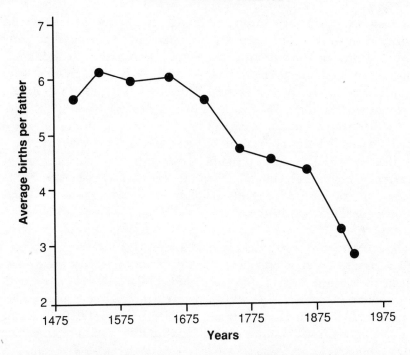

The declining birth-rates in European noble families. This evidence suggests that they deliberately limited the number of their children after 1700, possibly using interrupted coitus. There is not likely to be an economic reason for the decreasing fertility of the aristocracy.

contraception is an extremely ancient practice. The Petri papyrus, dating from around 1850 BC, describes how, in Egypt, crocodile dung was made into a paste and inserted into the vagina. The Ebers papyrus, probably dating from 1550 BC, contains a particularly interesting prescription: "Beginning of the recipes made for women in order to cause no conception for one year, two years or three years: Take tips of acacia. Mix with a measure of honey, moisten lint therewith and insert in her vulva." Of course, we have no idea whether this worked, but it is curious that the tips of the acacia plant contain gum arabic, and this, when moist and fermented, liberates lactic acid – a substance widely used in many modern spermicides.

Researchers have come up with some interesting evidence that contraception worked satisfactorily before the present century. For example, one study of Europe's ruling families showed that there was a

41

steady decline in their birthrate. Under scrutiny were the births to aristocrats in their first and only marriages. It was found that, from 1500 to the beginning of the 20th century, the number of children fell from a high of more than six (in about 1570) to about three.

Another study, which examined the birth rates of 1900 British aristocratic families, showed a similar trend: the mean number of sons fell from 5.6 during the years 1730–1779 to 2.4 during the period 1880–1939. As the only available methods of contraception were either abstention from sex or the withdrawal method (and, in the absence of contraception, abortion), it is likely that these aristocrats chose to withdraw. It seems unlikely, after all, that the average English duke would abstain . . .

The fertile period and temperature charting

The fertile period is, of course, the time in the menstrual cycle when you are most likely to conceive. Remarkably, it was only in the 20th century that people generally recognized the existence of a fertile period. The extraordinary studies of Dr Raciborski of Paris in the 1840s have already been described (p.22), but they did not gain wide acceptance.

The fertile period finally received attention after the turn of this century – not to help people to get pregnant, but rather as a method of contraception, advocated by birth control pioneers such as Margaret Sanger and Marie Stopes. Avoidance of the fertile period – the "rhythm method" – has been the only method of contraception that is acceptable to many religious groups, particularly Roman Catholics.

Timing the fertile period was virtually impossible until people became aware that a woman's body temperature rose after ovulation. Temperature charting was first suggested as a method of contraception in 1904 by a South African gynaecologist, Dr Van der Velde. The method for temperature charting is described on pages 110–11. While I am convinced that this is an extremely poor way for an infertile couple to time intercourse, I accept that this method may have limited use for normally fertile couples trying to achieve a pregnancy as rapidly as possible. Nevertheless, studies in the United States show that at least 20 per cent of women with a temperature that would be considered normal "ovulatory" are not, in fact, ovulating at all. And my impression is that at least another 20 per cent of women with a virtually flat or irregular temperature chart are ovulating normally.

Cervical mucus examination

As we have seen, cervical mucus changes in character during the menstrual cycle. Shortly after your period stops, the cervix begins to make watery mucus in increasing amounts. At the time of ovulation, this mucus production is at its peak and the mucus is at its most penetrable by sperm. It looks and feels rather like the uncooked white of a hen's egg. Immediately after ovulation, when you are no longer fertile, the mucus thickens and then shortly afterwards dries up almost completely.

Some women produce so much mucus at ovulation that it tends to run out of the vagina like a watery discharge; others produce very little. If you tend to have a clear watery discharge immediately before ovulation, you may have an obvious, simple external sign that tells you when you are ovulating.

Unfortunately, these signs are very vague in practice. If you have any vaginal infection (and this is extremely common), or if you have in the vagina any semen or other secretions from sexual activity, it is very hard to tell whether or not you are in a fertile period. Moreover, many women who are ovulating perfectly normally never produce enough mucus to make external assessment of this sort possible.

Urine tests for LH

You can now buy a kit from your local chemist which enables you to tell when ovulation is about to occur. This is a simple urine test, containing a chemical which changes colour if you are manufacturing plenty of the LH hormone. On the face of it, this seems a remarkable advance as it should mean that couples can easily decide when they want a pregnancy. Unfortunately, these kits are by no means all that the advertisements would have us believe. Several manufacturers are responsible for different versions of basically the same test and much glossy advertising and slick packaging has gone into them. I regret to say that I think they are almost useless as they have many serious drawbacks:

● The tests are expensive, costing perhaps £20–30 per month.
● Many people find it difficult to get the right colour change, and they get worried unnecessarily because they think they are not ovulating.
● The tests measure LH – the message to the ovary to ovulate. The ovary may get the signal from the brain but it may not respond. This is like your friend telephoning you at home – you may not be in to lift

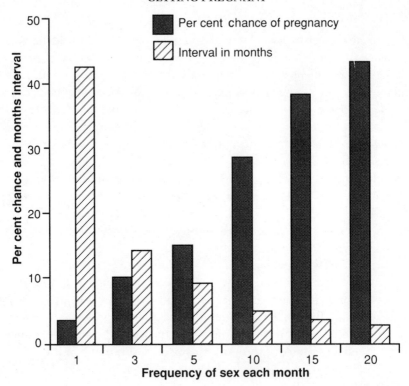

the receiver. This kit, in effect, merely shows that a signal went down the line, not whether it was picked up or acted upon.

● Some women have high, fluctuating LH levels which give false positive readings. They could think they are ovulating when they are not.

● The manufacturers imply that, by timing intercourse, you are more likely to get pregnant. This is debatable and, in my opinion, seems exploitative.

● Timing intercourse so precisely is emotionally destructive and can damage a relationship. In my view, it should be used with extreme caution by most couples, especially those who have already had difficulty in conceiving a child. It may be more satisfactory for a normally fertile couple, but then a normally fertile couple will hardly ever need to go to these lengths to get the woman pregnant. Consequently, I think these tests should probably be used only in very specific circumstances, and then probably under sensitive medical guidance.

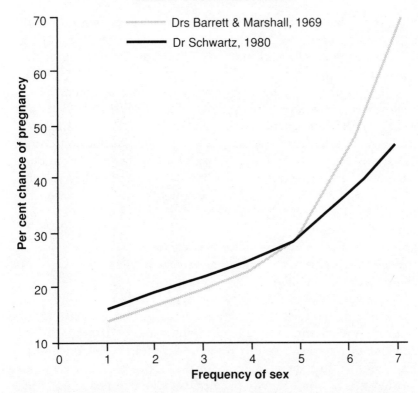

The chance of a normal couple having a baby depends very much on how often they have sex. Daily sex does not weaken the sperm; on the contrary, all the evidence suggests that fertility is improved with frequent intercourse. With sex once a month, the chance of a pregnancy is only 3 per cent, and the average time a couple would have to wait before conception is 42 months. With sex twenty times a month, the chance of conception each month is over 40 per cent.

Making love

I now can reveal how to get pregnant. No matter how many books you read on the subject, you will seldom find it discussed. If you are unlucky enough to be having difficulty in conceiving, you will usually not be told the real secret. The truth is that, the more often you make love, the more likely you are to get pregnant. The more infrequently you have sex, the less likely you are to conceive.

There are numerous myths surrounding conception. Two of the most common are:

- If you are having trouble getting pregnant, you should make love less frequently so that the sperm have a chance to get stronger, more copious and/or more active.

● You are not getting pregnant because you are not pinpointing the moment of ovulation.

I know of no evidence to support either of those statements. There is, however, abundant evidence that frequency of sexual intercourse is directly related to chances of conception, and that the timing of intercourse only needs to be loosely over the fertile part of the month.

Various recent studies have shown the advantages of frequent intercourse and its effects on conception. One, published in 1983, showed that couples having sex once a month between the woman's periods took an average of 43 months to conceive; with sex three times a month, the average delay in conception was 15 months; ten times a month, the average delay was 5 months; and if a couple had sex more than 15 times a month, the average length of time it took to conceive was 3.5 months.

A very good friend of mine – whose name I cannot publish because she would be besieged for all kinds of advice – had great difficulty getting pregnant for a second time. She is a very determined lady. After many months of failing to conceive even though she and her husband tried to time intercourse for the "fertile period", she finally insisted that her unfortunate partner made love to her at least once every night for a month. She says he was a bit exhausted after this (which, incidentally, he denies completely – though he certainly played less football), but her daughter was born nine months later.

CHAPTER THREE

Discovering You Are Pregnant

Some women are certain that they can tell when they are pregnant virtually from the moment of conception. This is difficult to prove, and seems rather unlikely. The embryo is so tiny in the first week or so of its life that it is invisible to the naked eye. Moreover, it does not enter the womb until about the fifth day after ovulation. We do know, however, that, although the embryo is free-floating at this stage and in no way attached to its mother, it soon begins to produce chemical signals – hormones – which tell the lining of the uterus to prepare for its implantation. The embryo, still microscopic, starts to attach itself there about a week or so after fertilization – that is, about 21 or 22 days after the start of the last period in a woman with an average menstrual cycle. Implantation is accompanied by quite a complex reaction, so it is just possible that this fierce little chemical fire is detectable very early on.

Symptoms that suggest you may be pregnant

Even before you may have a strong suspicion that you are pregnant, you may experience some of the following symptoms.

Tiredness
Many women notice that they are much more tired than normal. Very often this means being sleepy in the mornings or feeling very thick-headed in the evening. Carrying out routine tasks often seems to involve remarkable effort. This tiredness may be felt very early on,

and it frequently disappears later on in pregnancy, some time around the 12th week. What causes this tiredness and lethargy is difficult to explain, but it is certainly true that an early developing pregnancy consumes some of the body's energy sources. Interestingly, a few women feel much more alert in early pregnancy.

Nausea and vomiting

Feeling nauseated, or actually being sick, is one of the most common symptoms of pregnancy. Classically, this feeling is at its most unpleasant first thing in the morning, and is made worse by rapid changes in posture – for example, getting out of bed. However, it is almost equally common to feel sick at other times of day, particularly in the evening. Nausea can often be controlled to some extent by regularly taking small bites to eat, particularly food with a relatively high carbohydrate content – for example, dry biscuits.

Generally, nausea occurs slightly later than tiredness. Feeling sick may be due to the outpouring of pregnancy hormone (human chorionic gonadotrophin), which starts to increase about 16 days after ovulation.

Breast tenderness

This occurs very frequently indeed, and may be felt very early on in pregnancy. Some women certainly experience this as the first definite sign each time they become pregnant. Although breast tenderness is also extremely common towards the start of a period, very often women only experience it when they are pregnant. Sometimes, the first sign may be nipples which feel very tingly or particularly sensitive. I also know of some women whose first symptom is that their bras don't fit – though typically, breast enlargement is a much later sign, by which time most know for certain that they are expecting.

Changes in appetite

These are very common. Some women become exceptionally hungry in early pregnancy. Others feel like eating unusual foods. The husband of one of my friends always knows when his wife is pregnant because she starts getting out of bed at 5.00 a.m. to make peanut butter sandwiches – something that, normally, she can't stand. Some women develop a peculiar taste in their mouths, which they often describe as "metallic". A few women have an overwhelming desire to eat certain non-foods – a condition known as *pica*. I have known patients who ate plaster from kitchen walls and lumps of coal.

Urinary frequency

It is quite common for women in early pregnancy to feel the need to empty their bladders much more frequently. This can occur well before the time that the uterus starts to enlarge, so it cannot be due to the bladder being moved from its normal position. Having to go to the toilet frequently may be due to a high level of the hormone progesterone in the blood, which tends to relax the gut and bladder muscles of the body.

Mood swings, headaches, weight changes

Some women just feel different – either elated or depressed – in very early pregnancy. It is quite common to be unexpectedly tearful, just as you may be before a period. Headache, or even migraine, is a very unpleasant symptom. If you are unfortunate enough to suffer from these in early pregnancy, it may be some consolation to know that they tend to disappear completely by the 12th or 13th week.

Some women also lose or gain an unusual amount of weight in the first three weeks of pregnancy.

No period

Of course, this is the most important symptom of pregnancy. If you normally have regular periods and your period is late by more than four days, it is most likely that you are pregnant. Loss of a period (*amenorrhoea*) can be due to a number of causes, but in women up to the age of 40, it is most commonly caused by being pregnant.

Sometimes you may just experience an unusual period. About one-third of women have some kind of bleeding in early pregnancy at or around the time when their periods would normally occur. A period which is much lighter than normal, or much shorter, or accompanied by fewer symptoms of discomfort are all quite typical of those that occur in early pregnancy.

Testing for your pregnancy

Until comparatively recently, testing for pregnancy required a hospital laboratory. The most common test, until the 1960s, involved injecting the woman's urine into a rabbit or a toad and waiting many hours before inspecting the ovaries. Nowadays – and good news for toads and rabbits – most family doctors, family planning clinics or chemists' shops will arrange a rapid chemical test for you. This detects the pregnancy hormone *human chorionic gonadotrophin* (HCG), which is produced by the embryo within seven days of fertilization and is detectable in urine within two and a half weeks or so. There is also a rapid, and highly sensitive, blood test for HCG which can be done by many hospitals. This can detect a pregnancy within 12 days of fertilization – before a period is even missed. However, this test is not widely used because it is relatively costly.

Many women now like to test themselves for an early pregnancy. There are several excellent kits on the market, which you can buy from the chemist. Although most are very accurate, none is quite as good as a test done in a hospital laboratory.

● *Predictor*. This is widely available at around £7.95 per kit. It is very accurate and can detect pregnancy, in some cases, as early as two days after a missed period. You collect a sample of your urine immediately upon getting out of bed in the morning, as this is when it will be most concentrated. You mix this with a reagent in a little tube, according to the instructions supplied with the kit. You then insert a special plastic indicator into your urine for a variable amount of time (30 minutes if your period is two days late; 5 minutes if it is more than five days late). The tip of the indicator will turn pink if you are pregnant. Two points to remember: You should never leave the indicator in for longer than 45 minutes, as the result may be inaccurate. Also, the test is designed for normal room temperature, and may not be quite so reliable in a freezing room.

● *Clearblue*. This kit is available at around £6.95 for two pregnancy tests in one kit. It claims to be able to tell whether you are pregnant within a day of missing your period. With this test, you urinate over the end of a plastic sampler, which is then inserted into two plastic wells in turn for 10 minutes. It is a bit more complicated than the Predictor test, and can involve more time. As soon as the sampler has been washed under a running tap of cold water, you examine it to see if it has turned deep blue. If so, you are pregnant. If it is only light blue, you will need to test again in a few days. Points to remember: You must use cold water to wash the indicator. You must examine it immediately you have washed it, comparing its colour with that supplied on a chart. It is only accurate with concentrated, "first thing in the morning" urine.

● *Clearblue One Step*. A more rapid test has recently been marketed which consists of only one step. It costs about £8.35 for two tests. You simply place a small absorbent sampler in your stream of urine, holding it there for five seconds. You then secure the end of the sampler in its plastic cap and examine two windows in the side of the sampler. A thin blue line appears in the bigger window if you are pregnant. This test is also said to be capable of detecting pregnancy on the first day of a missed period. One point to remember: You must hold the tip of the sampler downwards in the urine stream. I like this test. One of my patients recently sent me her plastic sampler, with the blue line in the window to prove she was pregnant after some tubal surgery I had done. She also sent me a rose on St Valentine's Day, which worried her husband.

All these tests are reputable but, of course, not cheap. All may be inaccurate if you are having hormone injections containing HCG – which may be used if you are prone to miscarriage, or have been having test-tube baby treatment. In these situations, you can get a false positive result. False negative results may also occur, so if you continue to feel pregnant after repeating a negative home test, you should certainly see your doctor.

When to see your doctor

If you had no difficulty in conceiving, and have had no particular gynaecological problems in the past, there is no need to rush to see your doctor. If you have had infertility treatment or previous miscarriages or an ectopic pregnancy (*see* Chapter 13), you should make an appointment as soon as you think you may be pregnant. This is so you can be checked to ensure that the pregnancy is developing normally and is in the right place.

Most women want to have their babies in hospital. If you do, you should arrange to see your family doctor to get a prompt referral. If you have had any previous difficulties in conceiving, the hospital may well want to do an ultrasound examination (*see* p. 225). This is partly to date the early pregnancy accurately, but also to reassure you that the baby is growing normally. You should also arrange to see your doctor early if you have any serious medical condition – such as diabetes, heart disease, asthma or a kidney complaint.

CHAPTER FOUR

So You Want to Select the Sex of Your Baby?

In Chapter 1, we looked at the chromosomes. We saw that the sperm and egg each contain 23 chromosomes. When the sperm and egg fuse, the resulting embryo cell has 46 chromosomes, made up into 23 pairs. This total is kept in all cells which divide from the first embryonic cell. One pair of chromosomes, which are rather smaller than the others, contain (among many others) the genes for determining sex. The female sex chromosome is called the X *chromosome*, the male the Y *chromosome*. All mature eggs contain only an X chromosome. Sperm, on the other hand, may have either a Y chromosome or an X chromosome. When the sperm enters the egg, the embryo which results will either have XX chromosomes, in which case it will be female, or XY chromosomes, in which case it will be male. There must be at least one X chromosome in every mammal's cell (except the sperm cells). This carries other essential genes which are necessary for all animal life. Because the sperm may contain either an X or Y chromosome, it is the man who indirectly dictates the sex of the baby.

Curiously, there are actually more male babies conceived than females. In an average population, for every 100 girls born, there are 106 boys. The reason for this is not entirely clear. As far as we know, the number of Y-bearing sperm in a man's semen is equal to the number of X-bearing sperm. Consequently, it is thought that an equal number of female embryos are conceived, but that more are lost because they do not implant properly in the uterus.

Ancient customs, old beliefs

Since very ancient times, people have wanted to know in advance the sex of their babies and to be able to influence it. Boys appear to have been favoured by the ancient Chinese, and an Egyptian manuscript of 2200 BC tells that a pregnant woman with a greenish hue to her face is certain to give birth to a son. In ancient India, physicians suggested that if a pregnant woman had a fresh, clear complexion and a rounded abdomen, or if her right eye was bigger than her left, or if her left breast showed more activity than her right, this foretold a boy. This belief was also prevalent in ancient Greece and Rome. The Greeks also thought that boys moved earlier in pregnancy, a folk belief that prevails to this day. Hippocrates thought that stronger seed from the man produced boys – and, as we shall see, perhaps he was not far from the truth. However, he also thought that a mother who developed freckles was more likely to produce girls.

Many ancients thought the side on which the man and woman lay during and after intercourse was important – right for a boy, left for a girl – a belief which interestingly persisted even in this country until the 20th century. For example, the Greek philosophers Anaxagoras and Parmenides both said (in the 5th century BC) that if a couple had sex with the man lying on his right side and the woman lay on her right side afterwards, a boy would be conceived. It was thought that a fusion of the "humours" from the right testicle and the right side of the abdomen would form a boy. Anaxagoras actually proposed the tying off of the left testicle to produce only boys. Remarkably, some French noblemen in the 17th century were actually persuaded to undergo this form of half-castration to ensure an heir, despite the fact that, 2,000 years earlier, Aristotle (384–322 BC) had pointed out that men with only one testicle were capable of producing either boys or girls. These French counts were either ill read, well hung or desperate. Other Frenchmen of the time, being less bold, merely favoured pinching their left groin at the crucial moment of pleasure.

The timing of intercourse was also thought to be important by some Greek philosophers. Empedocles (c.490–435 BC), who is credited with founding the first medical school, suggested that males could be produced by having sex during menstruation, because he thought ovulation occurred then. Aristotle, who showed so much remarkable intuition about so many things and was an undoubted master biologist, felt that the timing of intercourse was not important in determining the sex of a baby as it was possible to have twins of different sexes. He also (rightly) argued that the sex of a child depended on the man.

The great Jewish writing, the Talmud, which dates from about the 3rd century AD, has several references to methods for sex selection. In one part, Rabbi Isaac states: "If a woman emits her semen first, she bears a male child, if the man emits his semen first she bears a female child." ("Emitting semen" probably refers to orgasm.) In another part of the Talmud, it says that it is a vain thing to pray specifically for either a boy or a girl. It is interesting that the ethical arguments for and against sex selection were considered so long ago. Recent Jewish commentators on this discussion in the Talmud ha e suggested that having a male child is a reward for having assured that one's wife has her orgasm first.

Why select the sex of your baby?

Various reasons have been given for people wanting to select the sex of their babies. Studies conducted in recent years show that even in apparently civilized societies such as ours, boys are more desired than girls. In one American study, 1,500 married women under the age of 40 were questioned, and twice as many wanted boys than wanted girls. The reasons they gave for preferring a boy were: to please their husband; to carry on the family name and to provide a companion for their husband. Another study in the US in 1970 showed that the majority of American women wanted two children, with a boy first.

In countries with high population growth and low economic development, boys are much more in demand. This is partly due to the fact that boys are more likely to become bread-winners and will be capable of supporting their parents when they are old and infirm. Two doctors, working in Poona, India, quote a farmer from the Punjab: "You were trying to convince me as a poor man who could not support a family in 1960 that I should have no more sons. Now, you see, I have six sons and two daughters and I sit at home at leisure. They are grown up and bring me money. Now, you see, because of my large family, I am a rich man. " A lucky man, indeed.

It seems that there was huge aversion to female births in ancient civilizations. It was no accident that Pharaoh found that the most damaging thing he could do to the Hebrews was to throw all first-born male children into the Nile. That way, of course, he destroyed the providers and soldiers. As recently as 1885, the traveller Vambéry, returning from Asia Minor, quoted the Turks:

If a daughter is born to thee,
Better she should not live,
Better she should not be born, or, if born,
Better the funeral feast with the birth.

Some modern authors appear to believe that sex selection could answer urgent world problems of overcrowding. They claim that the ability to choose the sex of one's child, combined with adequate contraception, would ensure a male and thus reduce the need for larger families – and, by implication, unwanted girls. The moral aspect of these arguments will be dealt with later.

It seems to me that the only valid reason for sex selection is for couples who are at risk of transmitting a severe disease which is sex-linked – that is, only boys or (more rarely) only girls will suffer the effects of such a disease. Perhaps the best known of these is haemophilia; another is a very grave form of muscular dystrophy; and some types of severe mental defect are also X-linked, only affecting boys. There are, in all, about 200 diseases which are sex-linked; most, but not all, of them affect only boys. In this situation, it seems perfectly reasonable to ensure that any child that is born is female, if possible. Interestingly, this approach would not eliminate sex-linked diseases, as they are generally carried on the X chromosome. Carriers of these diseases are girls, and they, though not affected themselves, could pass on the disease to half of the boys to whom they gave birth.

Factors said to influence a baby's sex

Stress

It has been claimed that stress is capable of altering the chance of having a girl. Professor Hampe, a German, writing in 1862, noted that poor people in a particular town during hard times were more likely to have boys. Dr Ploss, an Austrian, noted in 1882 that, given unfavourable conditions, male births were more likely. Several authors have since claimed that following various European wars, there was an increase in the number of male births.

Water supplies and environmental pollution

Dr Lyster made many studies of the different rates of birth of males and females in various populations under different environmental conditions in the 1960s and 1970s. He claimed that, in Australia, male births were reduced some 320 days after changes in the water supply, brought about by heavy storms. He also thought that a variety of environmental pollutants affected births – arsenic in the atmosphere causing an increase of males, births near iron and steel works being more likely to be female. Dr Lyster was a wonderful enthusiast, but his observations are not altogether accepted.

Seasonal incidence

In the last century, several authors claimed that more females were born in spring, more boys in autumn. Dr Dusing, a German who made many studies of factors affecting the sex ratio in the population, felt that the increase in sexual activity, due to rises in temperature, might play a part. Incidentally, I credit Dr Dusing with the first experiment to attempt to select sex in 1890. Because he felt that greater sex drive in the male produced a female baby (a widely held belief, dating back, as we have seen, to the Talmud), he tried an experiment in 30 cattle. He describes how he encouraged a bull to have repeated intercourse with many cows in order to weaken it. He then led the exhausted bull to a cow which was well nourished, well rested and sex starved. According to Dusing, because the cow enjoyed the subsequent conjugal relations with its tired mate, it produced a bull-calf. Conversely, Dusing claimed to have produced heifers by feeding a bull with plenty of good grass and isolating it from cows. In the meantime, its prospective mate had sex repeatedly with a castrated bull (so that it could not conceive) until the cow "no longer had any sexual desire". It was then mated with the well-fed but sexually frustrated bull. This procedure invariably produced cow-calves. Dr Dusing does not state whether he tried this approach in people.

Sex-selection methods of the past

Timing intercourse

Very many writers, since earliest times, have felt that the timing of intercourse (in relation to the time of ovulation) may affect the sex of a child. Various instructions are given in different literary sources.

The earliest detailed description I can find, which readers might like to try out, comes from an old Hindu source, the *Susrutas Ayur Vedas*. Assuming you want a boy, you must separate from your man three days after your period. A special, rich diet is recommended. On the fourth day of menstruation, dress in your best clothes and look at your husband. You should now avoid sex for one month, until your next period starts. Anoint yourself with oil on the fourth, sixth, tenth and twelfth nights of your menstrual cycle and make love. If you want a girl, try sex on the fifth, seventh, ninth and eleventh days of your cycle.

Some writers have claimed, until surprisingly recently, that women ovulate from alternate ovaries each month. This observation led Dr Dupuy (1888) to advise couples to count the number of menstrual periods since the last confinement. Those who wanted a child of the opposite sex from the previous pregnancy were advised to have sex only in the odd-numbered months following the last delivery (that is, to have a baby girl after a baby boy was born in December, intercourse should occur in January, March and so on). Looking back on the dates of my own children's birthdays, I found this theory to be totally proved.

Many modern authors have claimed that having sex close to ovulation is more likely to produce a girl. One study in Jerusalem, among very orthodox Jewish women who avoid sex for the first seven days after their periods showed that, in 3,658 births, 53.3 per cent were male if intercourse occurred two days before ovulation, 49.3 per cent were male if conceived on the day of ovulation and 65.5 per cent male if conceived two days later.

This method worked very well for Mrs Monteith Erskine, the wife of a Scottish MP, who in 1925 wrote a book, *Sex at Choice*, explaining how to get boys. She herself had conceived one girl and four boys precisely as she wished – depositing her secret formula for timing with her bankers in London. She also described how:

> ... Nature intended women to produce more boys than girls, and that, with this end in view:
> 1. She provided the girl-child with more male ova in her right organ ovary than female ova in her left.
> 2. She rendered easier the fertilisation of the right-side ovary ...
> 3. She made the right ovary and tube larger than the left and provided more seminal fluid for them to carry.

Presumably Mr Monteith Erskine was a Conservative MP.

More recently, various clinics performing artificial insemination using donor semen have had the opportunity to analyse their results following insemination at various times close to ovulation. A well-controlled study in the United States, showed that the sex of 1,188 children each conceived after a single insemination could not have been predicted by the time in the menstrual cycle when insemination was done. More recently, two doctors in London have found no evidence of a preponderance of boys or girls related to the timing of ovulation. They did find, however, that women who took clomiphene, the fertility drug, and who then had insemination appeared more likely to have girls. We have looked at women taking clomiphene in our hospital, and have not found any change in the normal sex ratio.

It is very likely, as we shall see later, that all these observed differences are due purely to chance. When the first test-tube babies were born, there was a definite increase in the number of girls – indeed, the first test-tube baby was Louise Brown and she had a sister a few years later, also conceived by *in vitro* fertilization treatment. Since then, however, the proportion of girls to boys has evened out. In our clinic, 52 per cent of these babies have been boys – what would be expected in a normal, untreated population.

Vaginal douching
Since about 1930, several doctors have claimed (without any hard evidence at all) that sperm with a Y chromosome prefer an alkaline environment, while X-carrying sperm prefer acid. They recommend douching the vagina with bicarbonate of soda for a boy, or vinegar for a girl. Apparently this should be done about 15 minutes before sexual intercourse. Try this if you must; my feeling is that your vinegar would be better employed on a green salad.

Shortening the odds
Dr Cedric Vear of Australia and Dr Landrum Shettles of the United States (both fairly controversial figures) have advised similar regimes, a combination of some of the techniques I have already mentioned, and have claimed that these work. If you have a good sense of humour, you might like to try to:

For a boy
1. Abstain from sex from menstruation until ovulation has occurred.

2. Douche with 5 g of baking soda in a pint of water, 15 minutes before sex.
3. Have sex with the man behind, and with deep penetration at ejaculation.
4. Ensure that female orgasm occurs before ejaculation.
5. Stop intercourse the moment the man ejaculates.
6. Repeat this rigmarole 2–3 times in the next 24 hours.

For a girl
1. Douche with 1–2 tablespoons of white vinegar in a pint of water, before sex.
2. Have frequent sex in the 7–10 days before ovulation.
3. Have no further sex during the 24 hours before ovulation is expected.
4. Have sex face-to-face, with only very shallow penetration.
5. Stop sex after ejaculation.
6. Ensure that female orgasm does not occur.

Using these techniques, Dr Vear had ten successes in ten pregnancies – but it took him seven years in a practice delivering over 100 babies each year. It is hardly surprising that he had so few volunteers when you think about it – a nice douche 15 minutes before intercourse, deep rear-entry sex with a good female orgasm, avoid sex completely for two weeks beforehand and then have it four times in rapid succession. I think he was quite lucky to find ten couples – how did he make sure they did it properly?

Diet
It has been suggested for well over 100 years that dietary factors can influence the sex of your child. Dr Schenk from Hamburg, writing in the last century, describes a woman who had five boys and who then developed diabetes; in her sixth and seventh pregnancies, she had a girl. Dr Schenk considered that her deteriorating body metabolism led her to have girls, and he "confirmed" this observation by studying the urine of many other patients – those that contained sugar were prone to give birth to girls. He therefore tried deliberately to reduce sugar in the urine with special diets to produce boys. One of his colleagues, in writing up these studies, remarked: "As is well known, Schenk was not altogether fortunate in his experiments."

Some authors have held that the mineral content of a woman's food can influence the sex of her child. Most of this work comes from France, a country where cuisine is noted for its powers. To obtain a boy, you need to have a diet rich in potassium with added salt. Such a diet might include sausage, meat, potatoes, beans, artichokes, peaches, apricots and bananas. For a girl, these foods should be avoided and more calcium with magnesium is needed. Suitable foods include dairy products, eggs, grapefruit, radishes, turnips and greens. A recent book by Labro and Papa (Photobooks, Bristol, 1984) describes the dietary requirements in detail. They do not look particularly appetizing to me and I am a little surprised that French pride allowed publication.

Getting your partner to change his job

One study suggests that fighter pilots have a 59.3 per cent chance of a boy, transport pilots 62.5 per cent and air field ground staff 60 per cent. Commercial underwater divers and anaesthetists are reported to have more girls. In practice, although various claims have been made, the variations in ratio can easily be attributed to chance.

Separating and selecting X- or Y-bearing sperm

It has been known for some time that male sperm are different from female sperm, and various scientists have tried hard to separate them. The idea is that, following separation, only sperm of the "right" sex might be inseminated into the woman's vagina. The X chromosome is a bit bigger than the Y chromosome, and therefore a female sperm might be expected to weigh very slightly more. A great deal of attention has been given to this, and several methods of separating male and female sperm depend on this rather obscure piece of biology. I calculate that a single sperm probably weighs less than 10 picograms (that is, ten million millionths of a gram). Regrettably the Y chromosome is almost the smallest identifiable structure in the sperm head, and at a liberal estimate an X-carrying sperm probably weighs no more than about 3 per cent more than a Y-carrying sperm. This is not much, not when dealing with such a minuscule object as a sperm.

Various laboratory methods for separation have been tried. They are all very similar, and all have similar deficiencies. The most publicized involves spinning semen in a centrifuge, having first suspended it in various liquids which have either a particular viscosity ("pourability"), causing more resistance to the sperm, or molecules of a certain size, which act as a kind of filter. Dr Ericsson of Sausalito, California, uses this method to separate Y sperm, saying that "it's like making them run the Boston Marathon with overshoes on". According to *Time* magazine, each clinic in the United States which uses his technique pays him $15,000 in franchise fees. However, Dr Sandra Carson, a reproduction expert at the University of Tennessee in Memphis, was unable to validate the method. Dr Ericsson's California car number plate is:- "x or y".

Does sperm separation really work?

Methods to separate sperm are not new. Indeed, an electrical method was first described by a Dr Schroeder in Germany in 1932, and since that time, it has been "rediscovered" by several authors. However, there are a number of criteria which have to be met before one can say that there is a genuine and reliable method for sex selection.

● *There must be controlled clinical trials.* This means that a given treatment, for which claims are made, has to be allocated to patients on a random basis in advance of treatment and the results assessed independently. So far, no method of sex selection has been subjected to controlled trials.

● *The observed difference between male or female births must be proved to be not due to chance.* Few methods of sex selection clearly demonstrate that the results they have produced are not due to coincidence. Hardly any of the authors have used a proper control group (i.e. couples giving birth who have not undergone any special treatment) to act as a simultaneous comparison, and most report very small numbers. For example, Dmowski, who used a layering technique in 1979, said that six out of eight couples had boys after his work. This ratio is likely to be due purely to chance. It has been calculated, using detailed mathematical formulae, that at least nine out of ten couples would have to achieve the desired sex before it could be assumed that the observed difference is not due to chance.

● *The method should be capable of such scrutiny that a reputable medical journal will publish the results, after independent peer review.* Authors of a substantial number of so-call scientific papers on the subject have not risked presenting their work to proper journals. In many cases, claims have only been made in the press – such as *Time* magazine.

- *Others must be able to reproduce the method both in animals and humans.* Very few, if any, of the methods of sex selection have been found to be repeatable by independent scientists or doctors.

What also impresses me about "sex selection" is that many of the methods have been promoted by fringe practitioners, and that some people conducting sex selection clinics seem to be making considerable sums of money.

A woman came to see me, complaining of infertility. Initially, she told me that she had been trying to get pregnant for two years, without success. However, she then revealed that she had already had three children, and that she had had no difficulty in conceiving each of them. There was nothing in her medical history to suggest why she should have become infertile, and her husband was in good health, she said. I was puzzled about her strange demeanour. When I hinted that I would much prefer to do tests on both her and her husband, she most reluctantly brought him to see me. It transpired that they had not had intercourse for two years. Eventually, I learned that all three of their children were girls and that they wanted a boy. Apparently they had been trying to conceive a boy by visiting an American practitioner. On three occasions, they had flown from London to New York, where a doctor there had inseminated her with her husband's sperm, having first treated it by a method of sperm separation. Each insemination cost $400 – a hefty sum considering that the laboratory work lasted 30 minutes and the insemination took 5 minutes. I suggested her "infertility" (which distressed her very greatly) was simply due to lack of having intercourse and that she might be better off trying to conceive naturally.

I can suggest an even better money-spinner for an enterprising young doctor. Human gullibility is such that it should be possible to offer a treatment for sex selection, with a full money-back guarantee. The doctor carries out treatment at $500 a time. If the baby is the wrong sex, a full refund would be made. This should offer a very attractive income, on the grounds that 50 per cent of the time the doctor would get things right.

Abortion

Clearly, one way of ensuring a baby of the "right" sex is produced is to screen each pregnancy by chorion villus sampling or amniocentesis (*see* p. 224). If the baby is not the desired girl or boy, termination of the pregnancy can then be carried out. From time to time, gynaecologists in Britain are asked to carry out screening and (if desired) abortion by patients who simply want to select the sex of their children for purely social reasons. I do not know of any colleague who is prepared to do this, and most people view the idea with alarm and repugnance.

This does not always appear to be the establishment view in other countries. In 1982, in India, two physicians in Amritsar advertised amniocentesis at 16 weeks' pregnancy to detect daughters, and offered abortions. After protests by women's groups, the health minister announced that such abortions were not allowed. However, surprisingly, the issue did not end there, and it seems that the Indian government, which sees overpopulation as the country's main problem, does not actively discourage the practice. In India, it appears that successful research on how to conceive males would be welcome. A review of attitudes to this problem was published in 1986 by the International Sociological Association.

It might be thought that, in Western countries, there would be very serious concern at the idea of aborting a foetus of the "wrong" sex. However, one study done by psychologists in the United States showed that up to 40 per cent of the population did not consider it particularly worrying and men were less concerned than women.

Commercial aspects of sex selection

It seems that all aspects of human reproduction are very interesting to the media. A recent programme on British television discussed a sex-selection kit, on sale in American supermarkets for just $40. If you want a boy, you buy the blue box; if a girl is desired, the pink one is purchased. Each kit contains a thermometer (value $2.50) and some litmus paper (probable value 50 cents). It also contains information about various positions you should adopt during sexual intercourse (value incalculable). The television presenter concluded: "It's a bit worrying that this is on the market. It is not available in Britain." She could have added that there is absolutely no evidence that it works.

According to the *Guardian*, one American company marketing a kit called "Gender Choice" (price $45) claims to have tested it with 6,000 couples with an 85 per cent success rate. The company, Procare

Industries, based in Colorado, hoped to export it to Britain in 1986. It involves the use of daily vaginal swabs to predict the ovulation pattern; how this might help sex selection is not clear, but the president of the company, a certain Robert Marsik, said that the secret lies in the *precise timing and method of intercourse*. It is interesting that there have been no validated medical trials of this product (published in peer review journals). So far, in spite of threats, this product has not hit the UK market as far as I know. Perhaps Mr Marsik became aware that there is some medical evidence to show that delaying conception around the time of ovulation might theoretically lead to a woman having a chromosomally defective child (*see* p.222). Perhaps he was worried about lawsuits.

From time to time, there are press reports from Japan about sex selection. Both *Time* magazine and *New Scientist* recently carried stories about methods to separate X- and Y-bearing sperm, to produce either girls or boys. Dr Iizuka of Keio University, Tokyo, has apparently used the technique to produce girls in all six patients who volunteered – a number too small to justify any statistically verifiable efficacy. Nevertheless, the results brought a storm of criticism from Japanese ethicists and were extensively published in newspapers there. Apparently this technique has also been used by a Dr Sugiyama in 120 cases: 24 women conceived, and in 22 cases, girls were subsequently born.

Dr Sugiyama's success rate – 22 girls out of 24 conceptions – is certainly large enough to confirm a definite effect not due to chance. Consequently, many Western scientists and doctors find it extremely surprising that, years later, the only accounts of this technique have been in the popular press and it has not been refereed by a medical or scientific journal. Until that happens, we shall remain sceptical.

Argument for and against sex selection

Many sociologists and psychologists have debated the consequences of sex selection. Their conclusions are as follows:

ADVANTAGES	DISADVANTAGES
Avoids sex-linked disease	Might benefit rich people only
Boys/girls might feel especially "wanted"	Boys/girls might feel "unwanted"
	Inbalance of sexes in population
Balance of two-child family	Increase in conflict between sexes
Reduction in population in under-developed countries	Risk of eugenics (i.e. "master race")
Increases human genetic controls	Possible abuse by the State

The main argument against sex selection, and the one most frequently presented, is that there would automatically be a preponderance of boys in the population as most people would rather have boys than girls. However, various studies have shown that, at least in developed countries, the preference for boys is very slight. Most people questioned have maintained that they do not care which sex their children are. About 4 per cent would prefer a boy and about 3 per cent a girl. It is very unlikely that this could make much difference, if any, to the ratio of girls to boys in the population at large.

So is sex selection really possible?

The answer is yes. Research in our department at Hammersmith Hospital now suggests that totally reliable methods of sex selection will be available, perhaps within the next few months.

The research involves using test-tube baby methods to collect eggs and fertilize them outside the body. One single cell, quite invisible to the naked eye, is removed from the embryo while it is growing in the test tube, two days after fertilization. The removed cell is immediately destroyed and its content of DNA analysed, while the embryo is kept in culture. Using a recently discovered method of gene amplification, powerful techniques are used to identify whether or not the single cell contains a Y chromosome. This test is so exquisitively sensitive that laboratory workers of the opposite sex to the embryo, by coughing carelessly or brushing cells from their fingertips, could introduce their own DNA into the solutions which are used and this could give a false result. However, so far, using absolutely strict controls, the sexing of each embryo has been done correctly. This technique is complex and expensive, and because of this it is inappropriate to be used for frivolous reasons. It has only been developed to help couples who are at risk of giving birth to children with serious or fatal sex-linked diseases.

CHAPTER FIVE

Late Motherhood

I find it very curious that we doctors regard pregnancy in a woman over the age of 30 as abnormal. Yet when I was in training, any woman having her first baby when she was over 30 was called an "elderly primigravida". This term seems to imply that the unfortunate woman is in her dotage and needs special mollycoddling to coax her through what is an appallingly dangerous time. It is perfectly true, of course, that biologically speaking the best time to get pregnant is between the ages of 20 and 25. However, in my own antenatal clinic the great majority of women are clearly "elderly", with an average age of over 35. This is because the majority of my own patients are rather infertile and usually have been trying to get pregnant for many years. They are none the worse off for that, and as they are all unfortunately younger than I am, I can hardly regard them as elderly.

Why are people waiting so long to have babies?

Perhaps the most common reason is simply that both men and women do not like to commit themselves early in life. In past years, people got married at a very young (perhaps too young) age. The changing pattern of Western society has meant that many men and women put off a firm commitment until much later, preferring to rear children when they are more sure of their own future. I think that, in many ways, we have become a very responsible society; I get the strong impression that a great number of men and women defer having children until they are certain of themselves as people, until they are fully mature.

Of course, while nowadays relatively secure and easy contraception has encouraged more people to delay childbearing, it is clear that a major factor is the question of career. Far more women than ever before work for a living. The gradual liberation of and increasing opportunities for women have also meant that they are faced with a dilemma. Many patients that I see have decided to establish themselves in a career first, before trying for a baby and then panic quite suddenly, seeking help to have a baby "before it is too late". Increasingly frequently we find that women over 30 who are having a baby for the first time are not married.

How age affects fertility

It is surprisingly difficult to prove that older people, and especially women, are much less fertile than younger ones. None the less, there can be no doubt that human fertility declines with age, and that, in women, this decline starts well before the menopause. This decrease is seen in all populations, in many different countries. In order to understand the way this opinion can be arrived at, and what its consequences are for the average couple, let us look at some statistics.

If we examine official records taken from all women resident in England and Wales in 1975, we find that there were about 690,000 pregnancies. This figure rose steadily over the years until, in 1985, there were 797,000 pregnancies. Incidentally, the number of pregnancies outside wedlock – 160,000 in 1975 – rose to 283,000 in 1985. Of course, not all these pregnancies resulted in children being born and many more occurred but miscarried, but these are not recorded in official statistics; in addition, 106,000 were terminated by legal abortion in 1975 and 142,000 in 1985. Fortunately, for our purposes, the Office of Population Census Studies gives a breakdown of the number of babies born to mothers of different ages (*see* p. 68).

What these figures show us is that only 4,800 women in England and Wales gave birth at or after the age of 40, both in 1976 and 1986. Although there was generally a trend for women to have babies at an older age – more women delivered a baby between the ages of 29 and 39 in 1986 than in 1976 – there was no increase in the number of babies born to women over 40. This suggests that, despite social pressures and trends, it was not possible for women to alter their basic lack of fertility after a certain age.

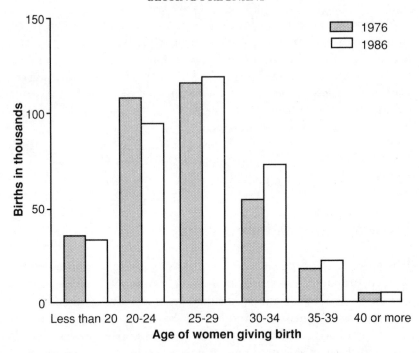

The statistics for births in England and Wales in 1976 and 1986.

If you are trying desperately to conceive and you are in the older age group, you might argue that the birth rates for present-day England and Wales are not truly representative of basic fertility because so many women nowadays use some form of contraception. For this reason, I have chosen to look at some statistics from populations who had no access to birth control. In 1985, Professor Trussell of Princeton University and Dr Wilson of the London School of Economics published an interesting study of British parish registers during the period between 1550–1849. In all, they looked at 16 different parishes, deliberately sampling a cross-section of the population of England to include rural villages, market towns, cities and industrial areas. They were examining how many women, married at different ages, did not subsequently produce children. Their data are important for three basic reasons. First, contraception was not in use during the period in question. Second, it is most unlikely that abortion would have any major influence on their results. Third, by careful reading of baptismal, marriage and burial registers, they were able

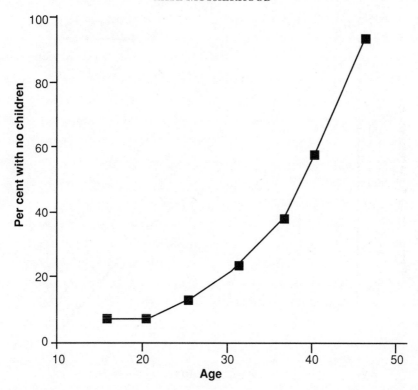

The chance of older women not having a baby.

to include only women who had "completed unions" – that is, those who remained married until the end of their reproductive period. Trussell and Wilson's results are shown in the graph above.

This fascinating study tells us a good deal about human fertility. We can see that only about 7 per cent of women who married at a very young age remained infertile but at least one-third of women who were married at the age of 35 did not give birth. Nearly 60 per cent of women married at 40 had no children, and there was only the tiniest chance of a pregnancy after the age of 44.

Is the phenomenon of decreasing fertility simply a British one? The answer is almost certainly no. Similar trends are seen in other human populations. Of particular interest are the Hutterite women. The Hutterites are an ultra-religious, in-bred, Protestant sect living in the United States and Canada. They have been repeatedly studied by anthropologists, sociologists and others for a number of reasons, one of

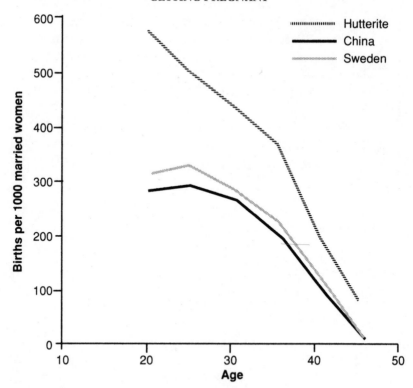

Declining fertility in three different populations.

the main ones being the Hutterites' high natural fertility: they seem to be more fertile than almost any other group of humans. Do they show a similar trend of decreasing fertility? Studies by Dr Henry (1961) and Dr Leridon (1975), illustrated above, confirm that they do.

Why are older women so infertile?

Like so many things about human reproduction, it is not fully understood why older women are so infertile. It is likely that several possibilities may contribute to the problem.

Decrease in love-making

It has been widely thought that infertility in older people may be due, at least in part, to a decrease in the frequency of love-making. We have already seen (p.45) that the more often you have sex, the more likely you are to conceive. All available sociological evidence suggests that the older people are, the less sexually active they become. However, hard evidence is not too easy to come by. Many questionnaires have been devised, but researchers never know for certain whether people responding to them have been truthful. Moreover, people often over- or under-estimate the frequency of their sexual relations. In addition, the frequency of love-making seems to vary from country to country. Professor Leridon of Paris has collected data from several studies; his results can be seen in the table below.

Monthly frequency of sexual intercourse by age of woman (only married women living with husband included)

Age of women	US	France	Punjab	Britain	Australia
16–20	11.0	–	8.5	9.9	17.2
20–24	10.1	10.9	8.5	8.2	12.0
25–29	9.0	10.9	8.5	6.9	10.0
30–34	8.0	–	5.2	5.3	9.2
35–39	6.8	7.8	3.0	5.5	8.0
40–44	5.9	7.8	2.2	–	6.8
over 45	–	3.2	1.5	–	5.2

Those who thought that the French were the sexiest nation in the world are clearly wrong. The British do no more than live up to other people's expectations. Australian women come up trumps, or perhaps they just boast a lot. Unfortunately, I know of no data suggesting whether Australian women are more fertile than others; however, Americans appear to be more sexually active than the British and this could explain why they seem to be more fertile. However, these data all confirm that sexual activity decreases with age.

Abnormal menstrual cycles

It is widely accepted that, as woman get older, they do not ovulate as frequently and that there are other abnormalities of the menstrual cycle which suggest a hormonal imbalance. There are two good studies – one carried out by Dr Dorling in 1969 and the other by Dr Vollman in 1977 – which confirm this (*see* p. 72).

These figures, while demonstrating that a sizeable minority of women have menstrual problems, also show that many have perfectly good cycles well into their late 40s. Clearly, then, failure to ovulate is

Frequency of abnormal cycles – irregular or anovulatory (i.e. when ovulation does not occur) – in older women

Approximate age	Abnormal cycles (Dorling's data)	Abnormal cycles (Vollman's data)
30–35	16%	13%
36–40	19%	11%
41–45	30%	16%
46–50	51%	30%

by no means the whole reason for failure to conceive in this age group. This is important because so many of the women of this age who come to me complaining of infertility are convinced that, because they are having normal cycles and are ovulating, they should be able to get pregnant easily. In fact, other statistics show that, on average, biological infertility commences ten years before the menopause (when periods stop or become irregular) in British women. What this means is that a woman has to put up with periods for an average of 10 years even though she has ceased to be fertile.

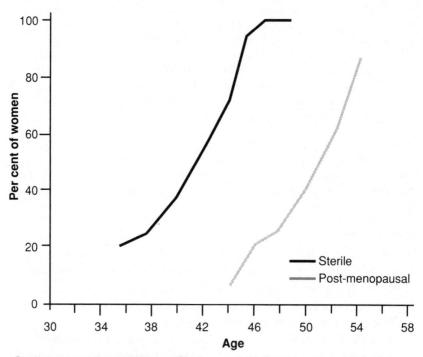

On average, biological sterility occurs about ten years before a woman stops seeing her periods.

Decrease in male fertility

A third reason is perhaps due to male infertility. There is quite good evidence that men, too, become increasingly infertile with age. Clearly, older women will generally be married to older men, and if it is true that male fertility decreases with age, this could partially account for the fact that older women conceive less readily.

Of course, male fertility does not decline as sharply as does female fertility – there is no menopause, as such. Moreover, it is true that many men remain fertile until very late in life. One of our husbands at Hammersmith fathered quadruplets at the age of 70. Pablo Picasso fathered a child at 80. One of the best examples of male fertility in old age is Baron Baravicino de Capelis of the Tyrol, who died in 1770. He married his fourth wife when he was 84 and had eight children by her – she was pregnant with the last when he died. His generative ability has been attributed to his diet – eggs, no meat, sweet tea and a cordial made to his own secret recipe.

There is, however, a serious side to the fertility of older men. Some recent research in Canada suggests that, compared with younger men, those over 45 produce far more sperm which are defective. It seems likely that at least 16 per cent of sperm from male Canadians over 45 have abnormal chromosomes, compared with about 4 per cent in men in their 20s. The precise significance of this is not clear. It could just account for an increased risk of abnormal babies, but may also help to explain why older couples are less fertile.

Increased risk of miscarriage and genetic defects

Older women have a greatly increased chance of miscarriage. Many of these lost pregnancies undoubtedly occur so soon after conception that women do not know that they have even been pregnant. Obviously, this may be a factor in the low fertility of older women. (For a full discussion of miscarriage, *see* Chapter 13 .)

Miscarriage at any age is extremely common. A study carried out in 1962 suggests that at least 23 per cent of all pregnancies of more than four weeks end in miscarriage. Another piece of research in 1970 suggested that 49 per cent of all fertilized eggs perish before full-time delivery. Results from patients having test-tube baby treatment (IVF) in our clinic suggest that the first figure may be a little high; we find that less then 15 per cent of test-tube pregnancies end in miscarriage once they have survived as long as four weeks. However, the situation following this treatment may be different from what happens

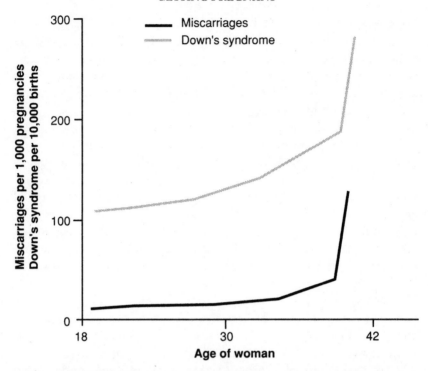

The rising incidence of miscarriage with age exactly parallels the rising incidence of Down's syndrome. This is evidence that faulty eggs are likely to be a common cause.

after natural fertilization – after all, following IVF only the best embryos are transferred to the womb. I certainly think it likely that at least 50 per cent of fertilized eggs do not make viable babies. What is clear is that older women have a much greater risk of miscarriage.

We do not know why the risk of miscarriage increases with age. Probably it is because an older woman produces less healthy eggs. These eggs have been held in her ovaries for a long time; indeed, they have been there since before her birth. Since that time, the eggs have been in arrested stage of development, and have been exposed to many potentially adverse influences in the environment. Eggs which have become damaged are more likely to produce damaged embryos if fertilized. This could well explain, at least in part, why older women are more likely to miscarry and also why certain genetic defects are more common in babies conceived by them.

We know that about about 40–60 per cent of all miscarried foetus show some chromosomal defect on examination, the majority being due to having one extra chromosome, medically called *trisomy*. It is worth remembering that Down's syndrome (or mongolism) is particularly common in pregnancies in older women. This defect is a trisomy, which fits well with this theory. What is even more interesting is that the increased likelihood of Down's syndrome with age closely parallels the rising chance of miscarriage. This, I think, gives us an important clue as to the cause of miscarriage in older women.

Problems in the uterus

Failure to get pregnant at a later age may also be partly due to problems in the uterus (womb), which in older women contains more fibrous tissue and less muscle, and is also more apt to contain a fibroid (*see* p.70) or have some adenomyosis (*see* p.155). In addition, the endometrium, its lining, is more likely to be abnormal and less able to help an embryo to implant properly.

It has also been suggested that the blood supply of the uterus is not as good in older women. The evidence for this is not yet very compelling, and more research is required. However, it could be one reason why infertility is more likely and miscarriage more common.

Do I run any extra risks if I become pregnant after the age of 35?

Being pregnant when you are older than average carries no very great risks. The great majority of "older women", when they are fortunate enough to get pregnant, have a perfectly healthy and happy pregnancy, a normal delivery and a bouncing, normal baby. The risks of pregnancy in older women can also be greatly diminished.

General medical ailments

All men and women are prone to ill health with age. All of us tend to be fitter at 20 than at 30, and fitter at 30 than at 40. Apart from general physical fitness and well-being, general health problems also increase slightly as we reach the age of 40. The most important of these are changes in our blood vessels. Unfortunately, perhaps partly because of diet and environment, we humans are really quite prone to diseases of the circulation system as we get older.

In pregnancy, the most important problem is an increased risk of high blood pressure. A rise in blood pressure, when it occurs, is more likely in mid-pregnancy and can affect the baby. Babies of mothers with high blood pressure are more likely to have problems or to be small and of low birthweight. Consequently, women with high blood pressure (hypertension) may require much more rest in pregnancy, and, quite frequently, even hospital admission before delivery. Raised blood pressure is more likely if you have a family history of it (about which you can do nothing) or if you smoke, are overweight, are under stress or drink much alcohol – and you definitely can do something about these.

Two other quite common circulatory problems which are a bit more likely in older pregnant women are varicose veins and blood clots in veins (venous thrombosis). Neither of these is particularly serious. Varicose veins can be unsightly and make the legs ache, but usually all that is needed are more rest than average and support tights. Venous thrombosis are more common after delivery than before it, and cause pain and soreness. Support tights are also often helpful with this complaint, and occasionally drugs to thin the blood and stop it clotting readily (anti-coagulants) may be needed. These drugs can be given quite safely and without risk to a woman of bleeding excessively during the delivery of her baby.

Other medical problems which occur slightly more frequently in pregnancy are diabetes, gallstones, bronchitis, certain rare types of anaemia and, very infrequently, low thyroid gland activity. None of these is common (except possibly diabetes) and certainly none is sufficiently serious to warrant any real concern about getting pregnant. The risk of diabetes naturally worries older women who are pregnant, especially if there is a family history of the disease. This worry is natural, but most diabetic states in pregnancy are simply and easily controlled with diet alone and, occasionally, bedrest.

Fibroids

One of the most common problems in women over 35 is fibroids. People with fibroids are less fertile than average. It has been calculated that, by the time they are 40 years old, about one-third of all women have some fibroids, benign swellings in the uterus (*see* p. 153). They can be only the size of a grape, but may grow to be bigger than a grapefruit. Fibroids very seldom cause symptoms in non-pregnant women and during pregnancy they rarely cause difficulties.

Miscarriage and stillbirth

The most important risk is very early loss of the pregnancy. As we have seen, miscarriage is much more common in older women. The reasons are not entirely clear, but are probably the same reasons why women over 40 are so infertile. Older women have eggs of less good quality in their ovaries, many of which may result in defective embryos. These embryos may survive very early pregnancy but could not survive in the outside world. The uterine environment is also less satisfactory with advancing years, and the womb may simply reject the newly formed embryo. Finally, older women are generally married to older men and, as we have seen, older men produce sperm with a higher percentage of abnormalities. You may read, or be told, that older women have a greater risk of miscarriage and stillbirth. It is true that, as a general rule, babies born to women over 30 are at slightly greater risk. However, this fact has to be seen in context. Most older women who face the greatest risk come from very poor backgrounds, tend to have poor nutrition, cannot look after their health and smoke heavily. Very often they have had many pregnancies, and this, too, can sap their well-being. It is therefore very important to get the real risk into sensible perspective; it is much smaller than those around you – even midwives and doctors – will have you believe!

Genetic defects

Just as miscarriage is more probable because of defective eggs, genetic defects are also a little more common in the babies of older women. The most important of these problems is the chromosomal defect Down's syndrome. Down's syndrome is usually caused by there being three copies (instead of the normal pair) of chromosome 21. About 60 per cent of cases of Down's syndrome follow fertilization of abnormal eggs carrying extra chromosomes. This condition is also more common in women who have already conceived a Down's syndrome baby. The increasing risk of conceiving a baby with Down's syndrome is shown in the chart on page 78.

Having three copies of one chromosome is called *trisomy*. Trisomy of other chromosomes is also a bit more likely in older women – in particular, trisomy of chromosomes 13 to 18 and, more rarely, trisomy of sex chromosomes. Down's syndrome is especially important because it accounts for a large proportion of all mentally retarded infants (32 per cent in Britain); it is, by far, the most common cause. Unfortunately, children with Down's syndrome also frequently have other defects (such as heart problems) and are very prone to infection; as a result, they have a greatly shortened life expectancy. The implications of all this are discussed in Chapter 14.

Suffice it to say, Down's syndrome – as indeed all other foetal defects associated with age – is reliably detectable early in pregnancy.

Risk of chromosome abnormalities in the babies of older women

Age of woman	Risk of Down's syndrome chromosome defect	Risk of any chromosome defect
20	1 in 2,000	
25	1 in 1,205	1 in 527
30	1 in 885	1 in 476
35	1 in 365	1 in 204
37	1 in 225	
38	1 in 180	
39	1 in 140	
40	1 in 109	1 in 73
41	1 in 85	
42	1 in 70	
43	1 in 50	
44	1 in 40	
45	1 in 32	1 in 23

For discussion of the pros and cons of screening for these defects, and the special tests that can be done, see Chapter 14.

Smaller babies

Older women are a little more prone to having babies of a lower than average birthweight. This probably reflects the fact that they tend to have higher blood pressure, and that the uterus has a poorer blood flow. For this reason, most obstetricians tend to want see older patients more frequently during pregnancy and may recommend rather more frequent ultrasound scanning. If your baby is growing at a lower pace than normal, you may be advised to come into hospital for a bit of extra bedrest and for monitoring of the pregnancy.

Problems during labour

Some older patients may have a bit more difficulty with delivery. My own feeling is that these difficulties are often greatly exaggerated. Positive thinking is better than negatively assuming that you will have trouble. It is true to say that if you are in the older age group, you will probably not be as used to physical exercise and, as a result, pushing the baby out may be more of an effort. However, your mental attitude is all important.

Fortunately, nowadays, getting proper help with delivery if you are tired carries no extra risk to your baby. If your baby is also getting tired or distressed, your doctor may want to do a Caesarean section. This may come as a shock initially, but it is worth remembering that it is recommended only if it is needed to ensure that your baby will be born with the least risk. Modern practice at many hospitals allows for you to have a Caesarean under local (epidural) anaesthesia, which means that you may be awake to experience the birth. In addition, it is increasingly common for partners to be together during a Caesarean section, and many couples find this a great comfort. If you are interested in this idea, it is well worth asking if this may be possible in your case.

Will I feel too old?

Perhaps the biggest problem that older women face is being afraid of feeling old. When you attend an antenatal clinic, you will be surrounded by women 15 or more years younger than yourself. This can give you something of a jolt. However, many more women are having babies later in life, and I know that in my antenatal clinic women find considerable comfort in meeting others who thought they were much too old to cope with pregnancy.

Some older women do feel more tired than their younger counterparts both during pregnancy and after it. Nearly all pregnant women get fatigued, and if you are older than average, you may need a bit more rest than usual. Very many women in this situation lose confidence in themselves and feel full of doubt. My own feeling is that, if you are fortunate enough to be pregnant at 40, you are privileged to be in a position of very special fulfilment and enjoyment.

Being older also has one other great advantage. You will be more experienced in life and more mature. This means that you will be able to be a bit more assertive than a younger woman in the average antenatal clinic. Don't be afraid to persist until you get clear explanations from your doctor and the midwives about what they have in mind for you. You will find it much easier to get information than many younger women. Being as old as (or even older than) some of the doctors and nurses can be a very great advantage.

PART II

If pregnancy doesn't happen

CHAPTER SIX

The Causes of Female Infertility

We humans are among the least fertile members of the animal kingdom. Even totally healthy women do not ovulate each menstrual cycle. Moreover, blocked Fallopian tubes or abnormalities of the womb are probably much more common in women than in animal species. And to make matters worse, the human male tends to produce more abnormal sperm.

In the past, it was widely supposed that infertility was a female "fault", and this belief resulted in a totally unreasonable burden being placed on many childless women. This depressingly chauvinistic attitude is still prevalent in some primitive societies, and regrettably, even in developed countries an irrational "female" stigma is widely attached to infertility. However, two things are clear. One is that infertility is only very seldom any person's "fault". Men and women, and particularly the latter, often believe that they are infertile because, in the past, they have done something that has led to the problem. However, as we shall see, this is very rarely true. The other thing that should be understood is that infertility is just as likely to be the man's problem as it is to be the woman's. Statistics show that only in about one-third of cases is the cause of infertility due to some failure of the woman's reproductive function; in another third, the man will be solely responsible. In the cases remaining, both partners contribute to the problem in some degree.

Few couples are worried if they do not conceive within a few months of trying. The gradual realization that there may be something wrong is often not talked about, but underneath people feel increasing anxiety. Usually, the woman takes the initiative by going to see the doctor, sometimes when her partner is not fully aware of her worries. Matters may come to a head when a couple find friends and relatives starting families without difficulty; and as they become increasingly aware that they have a problem, they frequently experience anger, frustration and, commonly a loss of self-esteem. Persistent infertility can be very corrosive, and if you have found yourself in this situation, you may well feel very sad and tearful. In particular, the grief of infertility often makes people feel guilty, as if they have actually caused their own problem. I have found that, if a man and a woman can find the reason for their infertility, it is very much easier to come to terms with the distress it causes – and it makes any treatment to overcome it much more likely to succeed.

Failure to ovulate

The most common reason why a woman may not be able conceive is a failure to ovulate. This accounts for about 30 per cent of female infertility. Fortunately, this is usually treatable by the use of fertility drugs (*see* Chapter 9). Why so many women fail to ovulate is not understood completely, but we know a number of reasons for it.

Hormonal problems

Sometimes there is a problem with the hormones secreted by the ovaries themselves, by the hypothalamus in the brain, by the pituitary gland at the base of the brain, or by the thyroid gland in the neck.

● *Failure to produce mature eggs.* In about half the cases of failure to ovulate, the ovaries do not regularly produce properly mature follicles in which the eggs can adequately develop. If they are not fully mature, it is unlikely that ovulation will occur, but even if it does, the eggs may fail to become fertilized. The most common disorder responsible for this is *polycystic ovary syndrome*, which may be caused by an imbalance between the hormones of the ovaries and those of the adrenal glands (just above the kidneys), or by an abnormality of the hypothalamus (*see below*).

● *Malfunction of the hypothalamus.* This is the part of the brain that sends signals to the pituitary gland, which in turn sends hormonal messages to the ovaries to cause them to produce mature eggs. In about 20 per cent of ovulation failure, malfunction of the hypothalamus is the basic cause.

● *Malfunction of the pituitary gland.* If the pituitary does not produce enough – or if it produces too much – of the ovary-stimulating hormones, the ovaries will be incapable of proper ovulation. This can happen if there is a chemical imbalance in the pituitary, or if it is physically injured.

● *Thyroid problems.* These are relatively rare, and require blood tests to identify them.

What to look out for

● *Infrequent periods*, occurring at longer than 36-day intervals. Occasionally there are no periods at all. Often your periods may be very scanty, with hardly any bleeding. However, some women who are not ovulating may have normal periods.

● *Weight gain.* Excess body fat is definitely associated with a failure to ovulate. If you think this may be your problem, you would be well advised to go on a sensible diet. Do not overdo it – losing too much weight can also cause infertility problems.

● *Excessive exercise.* There is now good evidence that repeated, vigorous exercise stops some women from ovulating. For example, running long distances every day may be harmful. If your periods are irregular, you may be well advised to cut down your physical training.

● *New excessive body and/or facial hair.* This is often a sign of polycystic ovaries.

Scarred ovaries

Physical damage to the ovaries can undoubtedly cause failure to ovulate. Sometimes the capsule of the ovary (its outer skin) can become so scarred after extensive, repeated surgery (perhaps for ovarian cysts) – particularly if this is also associated with infection – that the follicles cannot develop properly. This can be a side-effect of pelvis radiation therapy for cancer.

What to look out for

There is usually a medical history of multiple pelvic infections or repeated pelvic surgery, sometimes for the removal of cysts from one or both ovaries.

Premature menopause

A relatively uncommon cause of ovulatory failure is premature menopause, or premature ovarian failure. Some women, for reasons that are not well understood, seem to run out of eggs well before the usual age for the "change of life", and the level of the female hormone oestrogen in their blood is comparatively low. Menstruation stops completely, and menopausal symptoms such as hot flushes and dry vagina are common. The resulting infertility is usually not directly treatable, although hormone replacement therapy (HRT) will control the symptoms of premature menopause completely. Recently, however, childbearing has been made possible through *in vitro* fertilization: this is used to fertilize eggs from a donor woman, which are then implanted in the infertile woman, who goes on to have a successful pregnancy and delivery.

Premature menopause may be genetic. The condition certainly seems to run in families. In addition, there are certain genetic abnormalities that can result in girls being born with little or no ovarian tissue – *ovarian agenesis*. The most common is Turner's syndrome, caused by the absence of one of the female X chromosomes in all the cells of the body. Those who have this condition are usually shorter than average, and frequently have other problems as well, so that Turner's syndrome is almost always diagnosed well before puberty.

What to look out for
● *Complete loss of periods* or bleeding only at very infrequent intervals.
● *Hot flushes and/or dry vagina*
It is important to recognize, however, that these are very common symptoms and may not mean that a woman is not producing eggs.

Follicle problems
Some women appear to produce at monthly intervals a good follicle in which an egg develops, but for unknown reasons the follicle does not rupture on time and therefore the egg remains trapped inside the ovary. The mechanism behind this "unruptured follicle syndrome" is poorly understood, but it is receiving great attention from doctors in various parts of the world.

Psychological reasons
Most women, at some time during their lives, have a month or two when they do not ovulate. This most commonly occurs when they come under severe stress; during exams, after the loss of a job or the

death of someone close to them, during and after marital break-up, because of a bout of very bad depression. However, some women temporarily lose their ability to ovulate after far less traumatic emotional events.

Continued stress is only very rarely a cause of persistent failure to ovulate. This is why, in my view at least, it is unlikely that infertility is the result of psychological disturbance.

What to look out for

You may notice menstrual delay or irregularity, especially when you feel you are under stress.

Exposure to chemicals

The smoke from cigarettes is a common environmental chemical that may cause ovulation problems. Although many women who smoke heavily ovulate completely normally, smoking might interfere with good egg production.

Damaged Fallopian tubes

Fortunately, tubal damage seldom harms a woman's general health, and because of this, doctors believe that there is hardly ever any justification for treatment unless pregnancy is desired. As we shall see later, the most effective form of treatment is tubal microsurgery.

There are a number of causes of tubal damage, the most common of which is some kind of pelvic infection.

Inflammation associated with infection

There are a large number of different micro-organisms – bacteria, viruses and others – which can cause tubal scarring among other damage. For reasons which are not clear, some women seem to be more susceptible than others to infection by these sorts of microbes. It is often thought that tubal infection – or *salpingitis*, to give it its proper medical name – is always the result of promiscuity leading to sexually transmitted disease (formerly called venereal disease). This is, however, definitely untrue. Although salpingitis is rare for virgins and is more common in women who have regular sexual intercourse, it is now clear that it can be caused by many micro-organisms that are naturally found in the body, including *E. coli*, found in the bowel, and various forms of *Streptococci*, often in the vagina of perfectly fertile women.

However, the sexual pathway cannot be completely ruled out. Gonorrhoea is a major sexually transmitted disease that can cause salpingitis, and *Chlamydia*, micro-organisms halfway between bacteria and viruses, accounting for perhaps 15 per cent of all tubal damage, may be transmitted by sexual contact.

If you are unfortunate to have tubal damage, caused by an infection, you are likely to ask yourself how you caught the infection and whether your partner was responsible. Many of my patients finally bring themselves to ask me whether I think that they have caught a tubal infection from their husbands or boyfriends. The answer is almost invariably "No". Detailed research at our clinic a few years ago showed that perhaps no more than 10 per cent of women with tubal damage had definitely had a sexually transmitted infection.

Inflammation associated with abdominal disease
The most important of these diseases is appendicitis, especially if there is also peritonitis (a generalized infection of the abdominal cavity caused, in this case, by a burst appendix), but some forms of colitis (a bowel condition) may also be responsible. Inflammation of the abdominal cavity or the bowel can spread to involve the Fallopian tubes, which subsequently become scarred and blocked. Fortunately, although appendicitis is very common, it only rarely results in the tubes being damaged.

Inflammation following childbirth, miscarriage or abortion
The womb and the tubes are particularly susceptible to infection immediately after pregnancy. This is slightly more likely if delivery of a baby has been complicated – for example, if it has been a forceps delivery. After miscarriage, it is more apt to occur if an operation had been needed to remove all the tissue.

In the past – and today in countries where therapeutic abortions are illegal – backstreet, hastily conducted illegal terminations of pregnancy led very frequently to serious infertility afterwards. This is now rare in most developed countries, largely because abortions can be performed without any serious health risk. Nevertheless, it is extremely common for infertile women to wonder whether it is because they once had a termination that they are infertile now.

If you are in this unfortunate situation, it is hardly surprising that you might feel that you have brought this all on yourself – no matter how irrational this belief may be. Guilt about the past is quite a common emotion, but things should be kept in perspective. Remember that the vast majority of the hundreds of thousands of women who have abortions every year have decided that this is the best course of action for them – just as you decided that it was for you. The evidence is that a past abortion only rarely causes a present problem. You, and your partner, should try to draw a firm line across the past and look positively at what may be occurring now. If this proves difficult, counselling can be extremely helpful.

Surgical damage

A most important cause of tubal disease – and subsequent damage – is previous abdominal or pelvic surgery, particularly an operation on the uterus, Fallopian tubes or ovaries. Such operations, especially if they are done without a microscope (i.e. using conventional rather than microsurgical techniques), can lead to the formation of adhesions that may "glue" the tubes down so that eggs cannot travel through them.

Ectopic pregnancy

A pregnancy that occurs in one or other tube (*see* Chapter 13) often leads to scarring, which can cause tubal damage. Conversely and more importantly, tubal damage can lead to ectopic pregnancy.

Congenital defect

A few women are born with an abnormality of one or both tubes. This may also be associated with abnormalities of the uterus (*see below*).

Endometriosis

Endometriosis is a condition where the lining of the womb, the endometrium, grows not only inside the uterus but also in the abdomen. Occasionally, it can lead to severe scarring of the tubes or adhesion formation.

What to look out for

In most cases, women with tubal damage are completely free of any symptoms. However, there may be:

88

- quite severe period pains, or pain on intercourse.
- a history of pelvic infection, cystitis-like episodes that were never properly diagnosed, or a burst appendix.

An abnormal uterus

Problems in the womb itself account for at least 10 per cent of all cases of female infertility, but despite this, testing to see if the uterus is abnormal is often not done. This is a source of amazement to me – after all, the sperm have to pass through the uterus on their way to fertilize the egg, and the developing baby implants and grows there.

Fibroids

These are very common, benign (non-cancerous) tumours that can grow in almost any part of the womb. Many women who have them are completely fertile, and it may be that infertility occurs only when they grow in particular places – in the uterine cavity, or so that they block the Fallopian tubes or dislodge the ovaries from their normal position.

Why they grow at all is a total mystery. We do know that they are much more common in women over the age of 35 and that they do not develop after the menopause. There also seems to be a genetic predisposition to fibroids: they often affect more than one female member of a family, and certain racial groups – such as black African women – are more prone to them. However, fibroids are so common that about one in every 3 women will have some by the age of 40. This may sound a little frightening, but it is rare for fibroids to cause any serious problems – apart, that is, from infertility.

What to look for
- Increasing heavy and painful periods.
- Swelling in the abdomen.
Many other conditions can also cause these very common symptoms, but infertility may be the only sign that something is wrong.

Adenomyosis

This condition is perhaps rather more common than is often thought. Normally the lining of the uterus – the endometrium – is shed about once a month at menstruation. However, in adenomyosis, part of the lining grows into the thick muscle of the uterus and, consequently, some menstrual bleeding occurs there. Usually only isolated areas are affected, but occasionally the whole of the uterine muscle wall is involved.

The uterine lining can also grow into a Fallopian tube at the point where it meets the uterus. This can cause sufficient scarring to block the tube partially or completely. However, whether or not the tubes are blocked, adenomyosis is commonly associated with infertility.

What to look for
- Prolonged, painful periods; often the pain is dull and continuous.
- Occasionally the womb may be enlarged and a bit tender.
- Dull pain on intercourse.

Congenital abnormalities

A surprising number of perfectly healthy women are born with an abnormality of the uterus. In many cases, this does not cause infertility, and they may go through life without knowing that their uteruses are any different from anybody else's.

In all mammals – rabbits, cats, dogs, sheep, whales, monkeys, humans – the uterus develops from two separate tubes in the abdomen of the embryo, one on the right side of the body and the other on the left. In monkeys and humans, these two tubes become fused together to form one cavity with one womb. However, virtually all other mammals develop two separate wombs on either side of the abdomen.

Because the human uterus grows from the two tubes fusing together, most abnormalities result from incomplete fusion. In some cases, the embryonic tubes fail to stick together at all, resulting in the woman having two uteruses, both smaller than one fused uterus. This may cause infertility and, not infrequently, recurrent miscarriages. Much more common, however, is a *septate uterus* – a protrusion into the upper part of the uterine cavity. This may cause no problems, but it is known to be associated with miscarriage, rather than an inability to conceive.

As well as problems with conception and miscarriage, these abnormalities can sometimes cause unusually painful periods. They may also lead to problems during childbirth – for example, the baby may lie in the breech position, or there may be trouble delivering the placenta at the end of labour.

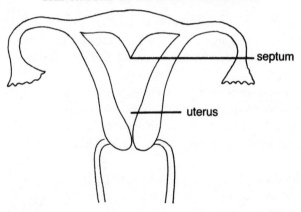

A septate uterus, a common cause of both infertility and miscarriages. Although the inside of the uterus is very indented by the septum, note that outside it has a normal contour. A septate uterus may therefore not be apparent on laparoscopy alone, and X-ray is usually essential.

Uterine adhesions

About half of the women with uterine problems that we see in our clinic have adhesions in the inside of the uterus. This means that the internal walls of the womb are stuck together, causing the cavity to be distorted. The problem usually follows a previous pregnancy – either one that ended in miscarriage or abortion or was completed but childbirth was medically complicated in some way.

This condition is frequently referred to as *Asherman's syndrome*, after Dr Asherman of Jerusalem who first described it in 1947. He felt that these adhesions nearly always followed physical trauma – usually injury to the walls of the uterus following a curettage ('scrape" or D&C) after a miscarriage or termination of pregnancy.

What to look for
● Periods that have become scanty or stop altogether following a miscarriage, abortion, difficult delivery or, occasionally, removal of a uterine fibroid (*myomectomy*).
● Painful cramps during periods, the pain usually starting when the flow is at its heaviest.

Polyps or foreign body in the uterus

Any solid object that intrudes into the uterine cavity may prevent a woman from becoming pregnant. Indeed, if you think about it, this is how the contraceptive coil (IUD) works.

Solid uterine objects are not that common. They include polyps – fleshy, grape-like growths of the uterine lining that are not shed – and small fibroids. Very occasionally, there may be a forgotten contraceptive coil, or part of one if it has been incompletely removed.

What to look for

There are often no symptoms. However, there may be painful cramps during periods, sometimes associated with heavy bleeding, and, occasionally, bleeding or spotting between periods.

Problems with the cervix

The cervix performs two vital functions in conception and pregnancy. First, it acts as an important reservoir for sperm. After sexual intercourse, the sperm stay in the cervical mucus, from where they swim up into the uterus and through into the Fallopian tubes to meet the egg.

Second, the cervix holds the uterus shut once you are pregnant so that the developing embryo and foetus are kept safely inside to develop completely.

Problems with the cervical mucus

There are several reasons why sperm may not survive in the cervical mucus. It may not be of good quality because hormone levels are wrong. Adequate amounts of watery mucus in which the sperm can swim easily are made in the cervix in response to the hormone oestrogen. Virtually the only time during the menstrual cycle when conditions are right for sperm is just before ovulation (this is why checking a condition of cervical mucus is used in some forms of birth control). Thick mucus, on the other hand, is made in response to the hormone *progesterone*, which is usually produced *after* ovulation. If your body is not producing enough oestrogen, the mucus may be scanty or very thick and the sperm may not be able to swim through it to reach the egg. The most common reason why insufficient oestrogen is produced is failure of ovulation (*see above*).

The secreting cells within the cervix may themselves be abnormal and incapable of making enough mucus. This sometimes happens after severe infections of the cervix, or if the cervix has become scarred. Some operations on the cervix may remove so much of its surface that mucus production is greatly reduced.

Finally, a woman may produce antibodies to sperm, which attack them in the cervical mucus. Antibodies are part of the body's defence against bacteria; they kill off harmful germs – or indeed any other foreign material, especially foreign proteins – which may cause you harm. Sometimes, however, this defence mechanism goes wrong, in which case you can produce antibodies against completely harmless substances. This can result in, among other things, certain forms of food allergies, sensitivity to cat fur, asthma attacks and so on. The same thing can happen in response to the presence of sperm.

Problems with the cervix itself

If the membranes surrounding the developing baby "pout" through the opening of a cervix that is abnormally widened, infection can set in, the membranes can rupture and miscarriage or early labour occurs. This disaster is, unfortunately, quite common. If you have had a miscarriage between 16 to 26 weeks after conception, it is possible that your cervix opened, or, to use the technical term, you may have an *incompetent cervix*.

Cervical incompetence may occur because of a congenital weakness in the muscles of the cervix. It can also follow injury – for example, if the cervix has been damaged during an operation to remove the remaining products of conception following a miscarriage, or during a complicated delivery or late abortion. Luckily, in the great majority of cases, this condition is easy to treat.

CHAPTER SEVEN

The Causes of Male Infertility

At least 30 per cent of infertility is due to a problem in the man. In spite of this, it is surprising how often the burden of infertility is borne by female partners. Most infertility specialists, for example, are gynaecologists – that is specialists in the medicine and surgery of the female reproductive system. Indeed, in Britain at least, there are very few *andrologists* (specialists in the male reproductive system). In many infertility clinics, the woman is often seen by herself and she alone is examined. The male is relegated to merely providing a sperm specimen. This traditional view of infertility is outmoded and wrong. In my view, wherever possible a couple should go together to a specialist, if they are seeking help.

Unfortunately, male infertility carries a stigma. Consequently, very many men are reluctant to have tests. When a woman is infertile, she quite often has some physical symptoms; she may therefore go to her doctor with some idea that her body isn't working normally. Male infertility seldom causes symptoms, and this is one reason why some men resist becoming involved with tests. This refusal can cause friction between a man and a woman, especially if there is a likelihood of there being a male problem.

Many men are much more distressed at being infertile than are their partners. Some become very disturbed indeed, or clinically depressed. For some men, finding out that their sperm count is low means that they are the responsible party – the guilty one. They have to live with a sense of loss and can, quite illogically, feel deeply ashamed. Male infertility is a condition which, by its very nature, usually hits a man between the ages of 25 and 45, just when he may be trying to establish himself in other ways – perhaps in a better job. Frequently the sense of failure spills over into other aspects of his life, such as failed professional ambitions.

Of course, a woman may be upset about her partner's infertility, but generally the extent of these feelings seems greater to her partner than they really are. She may indeed feel angry at being denied a child through no fault of her own, but this anger conflicts with her love and feeling for her partner so that she becomes very confused. Most women patients I know would much prefer the problem to be theirs; they feel that they would find it easier to deal with emotionally, fearing the effect that the diagnosis of subfertility or infertility will have on their partners. Often they resist the idea that their men should be tested, and try to shelter them. They may even go through all sorts of tests without even telling their partners that they are attending an infertility clinic. Other women find that their partners will not see a doctor at all, nor will they produce sperm for testing. These men neither want to go through the ordeal of the test nor want to admit to why they feel it is an adverse reflection on their sexuality.

It is quite common for people to think that they are inadequate sexually simply because they can't have children. Men feel this particularly. There is widespread confusion between infertility and sexual performance, virility and masculinity. In fact, there is no connection and a man's potency is in no way related to his ability to produce sperm. It is equally true that men who are impotent and unable to give their partners any pleasure at all through sexual intercourse are as likely as the rest of the population to be perfectly fertile.

These sexual feelings may present themselves in different ways in the doctor's consulting room. Sheila and Joseph, a very happily married couple, originally consulted us because they had been trying to get pregnant for seven years; before they were seen by us they had been told that there was no explanation for their infertility. Detailed testing in our clinic clearly showed that there was a real reason for the problem, namely that Joseph was mostly producing very abnormal sperm which were quite incapable of fertilizing eggs. Only a few of the sperm were normal, just sufficient for them to be considered for test-tube baby treatment (IVF). They were placed on the waiting list for this to be done, which at that time was about ten months long. Four months later, they came back to see me and asked for Sheila to have artificial insemination with Joseph's semen until the time came for IVF. I pointed out that insemination would be most unlikely to help and that natural intercourse was generally much more successful. At this point, Sheila burst into tears. It gradually came out that, since we had firmly established the cause of the infertility, Joseph had become completely impotent. It took a good deal of treatment and counselling before these sexual difficulties were resolved.

Why are some men infertile?

No sperm in the semen fluid

Occasionally no sperm are being produced in the semen. This may be because none is being made by the testicle, or because they are not being ejaculated during orgasm. Failure to ejaculate sperm in spite of their production by the testicle is due either to the tubes from the testicles to the seminal vesicles being blocked (*see* illustration on p. 25), or to the muscles that pump semen through the urethra not working properly.

It is rare for the testicles to fail to make any sperm at all. Fewer than 5 per cent of infertile men have this problem. Just as complete ovarian failure in women is usually untreatable, total failure of the testicle is very difficult to alter. Usually it is impossible to find the cause. It may be due to a hard blow to the testicles, such as a sporting injury, a previous severe mumps infection, or damage to the blood supply to the testicle, usually due to serious twisting of the testicles. If this is the case, the doctor may make the diagnosis easily from discussing the man's past medical history.

Testicular failure may also be due to a hormonal cause. The pituitary gland in the brain may not produce enough hormones to stimulate the testicles. Alternatively, the testicles may not respond to these hormones for several, mostly uncommon, reasons:

● The man's testicles did not descend into the scrotum after birth and they are usually not properly developed and cannot make sperm.
● The cells of the testicles are unable to make sperm even when there is enough male hormone.
● There is a rare defect from birth. This is likely to be chromosomal.

These three conditions are usually untreatable, although in rare cases, hormones may help.

If the minute tubes that connect the testicles to the seminal vesicles are blocked, the testicles may produce sperm but these cannot get into the semen. Blockage of these tubes is a result of scarring, sometimes due to an infection such as gonorrhoea or tuberculosis, or occasionally because of injury. Men may also be born with blockages of part of this system of tubes. Such blocks may be amenable to surgery.

In about 1 per cent of cases, the genital muscles do not pump in a properly coordinated way during orgasm. Sperm may enter the bladder and mix with the urine, rather than get into the woman's vagina. This is called *retrograde ejaculation* and may follow an operation such as the removal of the prostate gland. It may also happen if the nerves to the muscles are damaged. Some drugs, particularly tranquillizers and those used to control high blood pressure, may also temporarily cause this.

The semen contains few sperm

The vast majority of cases of male infertility (about 70 per cent) are due to a low sperm count. There are very many reasons for this, but most of the time the real cause cannot be established with any certainty. Regrettably, when the count is low, many of the sperm which are present in the semen are frequently either of poor motility (i.e. they do not move properly) or they are abnormal in some way (*see below*).

If the sperm count is low but the sperm themselves are quite normal, the outlook is good. Most men in this situation are very likely to get their partner pregnant eventually, though often it may take very much longer than normal for this happy outcome.

Sperm that are largely abnormal or of low motility

There are many reasons why sperm are abnormal, but in most cases a definite cause cannot be found. In many men, there is probably a genetic defect which accounts for this. Also, as a man gets older more of his sperm tend to be abnormal or of low motility. Some of the known causes include:

• *Hormonal problems* which may drastically reduce sperm quality. Generally, the more severe the hormonal problem, the worse will be the sperm motility or quality.

• *Abnormal blood vessels around the testicle* may be associated with "bad" sperm. There may be enlarged veins, rather like varicose veins, draining the testicles. This condition is known as *varicocoele* and is thought by some people to cause overheating of the testicles. The blood in the enlarged veins may indeed be keeping it at a higher temperature than normal, but this is almost certainly not the whole story (remember the elephant in Chapter 1?). The real reason why a varicocoele causes some men to be infertile but not others is not yet known.

● *An infection* that has lasted a long time is sometimes thought to cause poor sperm quality. An infection of the prostate gland may be found in a few men with poor sperm. Some doctors believe that one group of microbes – the *mycoplasmas* – are particularly likely to cause problems, perhaps by reducing sperm motility. The mycoplasmas have recently come under considerable scientific scrutiny. There is good evidence in animals that these organisms may interfere with the ability of sperm to fertilize an egg. Although these microbes are not at all dangerous to general health, antibiotics may be given in an attempt to improve the quality of the sperm.

Sometimes sperm that look normal under the microscope are actually chemically abnormal. This is not common, but is seldom treatable with drugs.

Immunological problems

About 5–10 per cent of male infertility is caused by an immune reaction. For reasons that are not yet known, some men form antibodies to their own sperm. The body "sees" the sperm as "foreign" and attacks them with its immune defences. This action is very similar to how the body protects itself from being invaded by foreign proteins, bacteria or cells. Unfortunately, in this situation it causes an unwanted consequence. Why antibodies occur is uncertain, but they may be a response to some kind of injury earlier in life.

Difficulty with intercourse

Difficulty with sexual intercourse is very rarely the cause of male infertility (less than 1 per cent). Sexual difficulties can result in sperm not being ejaculated into the vagina. The commonest problem is what is called *premature ejaculation*, when the man has his orgasm before he is able to get the penis deep into the vagina. This is more likely in very young men and can be overcome with patience and practice.

There are many other reasons for difficulty with intercourse, and these are outside the scope of this book. Sexual problems need specialized help, and the best people to consult are often counsellors trained in marriage guidance. Your family doctor can suggest the best sources of help. Although many men may, at first, feel too embarrassed to discuss this, sympathetic advice is readily available from those familiar with these problems.

Anatomical abnormalities

These are also very rare. The most common is the condition known as *hypospadias*, when the urethra (the tube running through the penis) opens into the outside world underneath the penis or even near the scrotum. As with retrograde ejaculation, sperm are not ejaculated into the vagina. This can be treated with a simple operation.

Absence of the vas deferens, or poorly developed testicles are other rare anatomical abnormalities that can affect fertility.

Environmental factors

Certain environmental factors contribute to reduced sperm production and poor sperm quality. Severe pressure of work, smoking and excessive alcohol all can result in a reduction of male fertility. This is very important as often these factors are very easily corrected (*see* pp. 128–30 for more discussion of this). There are a number of reasons why a man's sperm count can be depressed:

● *Smoking.* This may have no effect on many men with completely normal or high sperm counts. However, if a man is prone to underproduce sperm, he may have a catastrophic drop in sperm numbers and quality if he smokes.

● *Alcohol.* Like tobacco, alcohol is a poison, and it damages the cells which make sperm. In most men, heavy drinking over a period of time is likely to reduce their ability to make sperm. Different men have a different tolerance to alcohol, but it is certainly important for a man to restrict his drinking if he is prone to this problem.

● *Being overweight.* Although many obese men are fertile, there is an increased chance of infertility if a man is overweight.

● *Caffeine.* There is increasing evidence that both excessive coffee and tea drinking may be associated with both male and female infertility. In men, this is caused by sperm defects; the reason why it prevents women conceiving is not understood.

● *Drugs.* Several drugs reduce sperm count. On the list of "social" drugs is cannabis (marijuana): there is no doubt that this can have a powerful effect on the sperm of some men, and its use should be avoided. Medicinal drugs that may depress sperm count include:

Anti-depressants
Anti-malarial drugs
Anti-hypertensives (for treating high blood pressure)
Sulphasalazine (brand name Salazopyrin; used for colitis)
Cytotoxic drugs (for blood disorders and certain cancers)
Nitrofurantoin (brand name Furadantin; used for bladder
    infections)
Steroid drugs such as cortisone (this is not proven, but they may
    affect some men)

● *Excessive exercise.* Regular sport, jogging or cycling promotes
well-being, but there is evidence that excessive strenuous exercise
may affect sperm production. We know that some athletes at the
peak of training have reduced sperm counts, but these return to
normal when they exercise less and gain a little weight.

● *The stresses of work and daily life.* This is a most difficult factor to
weigh up. It is always a problem to understand just which aspects of
anyone's life may be contributing to poor fertility. At particular risk
are people such as the high-powered executive, who is constantly
flying around the world and is under pressure all the time. To make
matters worse, he may often be away from home for long periods,
perhaps at those times when his wife is most fertile. Apart from
reducing the chance of conception, time away from home throws
added strain on the sexual and marital relationship, compounding
stress. These professional pressures are often worst when a man is in
his 30s and early 40s, yet this may be the best time to have a child,
particularly as a woman's fertility is decreasing as time creeps on.
High rates of stress are also experienced by those in low-skill manual
jobs, such assembly workers.

● *Occupational hazards* Other occupations associated with sperm
problems include those involving long-distance driving or jobs where
there is exposure to poisonous substances such as lead – for example,
lead-laden petrol fumes in a bus depot. Men exposed to excessive
vibration, such as boiler makers or pneumatic drill operators, or
those in any other jobs where the environment is very tiring or
stressful, may also be affected.

Some people think the quality and quantity of their sperm may be
reduced if they have sex too often. This has not been proved, and I,
for one, don't believe it. We know that many men who have intercourse several times a day are completely fertile.

CHAPTER EIGHT

Investigating Infertility

It is crucial to understand that infertility is not a disease. It is a symptom that something is not quite right with one or even both of you. Before having treatment for infertility, it is essential that proper tests are carried out to find the cause. If this is not done, the wrong treatment may be given, with inevitable delays in solving your problem. For example, far too many women are given fertility pills when they first go to their doctor complaining of difficulty in conceiving. This is a mistake. First, not only might it delay finding the real cause of their trouble, which results in a delay in them getting effective treatment for the real cause, but inappropriate treatment may actually prevent conception. For example, clomiphene tablets (brand name Clomid, the most common fertility pill) can actually prevent women conceiving if they do not have a problem with ovulation.

When should you consider infertility test?

It is seldom worth worrying unless you have not conceived despite having had regular sex without contraception for at least six months. In couples where the woman is under 30, it is not unreasonable to wait two years before embarking on tests. If the woman is over 30, there is a bit more urgency. Obviously, if you are 30 or more you will naturally feel that time is running out. Here is a paradox: as the older woman tends to be a little less fertile anyway, she may naturally take longer to conceive. Nevertheless, if you are in this age group and you have not conceived after 12 months, I would recommend comprehensive tests.

You may want earlier investigation than I have recommended.

This may be because you have a good reason to believe that you have a definite problem. With any of the following symptoms, it might be silly to wait too long before tests are done:

History/symptoms	*Possible cause/result*
WOMAN	
No periods for some time	Probably not ovulating
Very infrequent periods	Not ovulating regularly
Painful periods *and* deep pain on sex	Inflammation or endometriosis
Recent very heavy periods	Problem in the uterus
Previous operation for ovarian cyst	Adhesions
Previous burst appendix	Tubal problems
History of infection with contraceptive coil	Adhesions
Previous infection immediately after pregnancy	Pelvic inflammation
MAN	
Mumps during adult life	Poor sperm production
Definite testicle injury	Poor sperm production

This list is not exhaustive, but it does contain the more common reasons for seeking early help. If you think you may have another problem, you should consult your family doctor, who will certainly be able to advise you on what to do.

Trying to ensure reasonably prompt diagnosis

Once you have decided on infertility tests, a diagnosis should usually be made well within six months. A few couples, especially younger ones, may decide to have a few simple tests and then await events. Generally, though, once you have started on tests, you are probably best to establish the cause (or causes) of the problem so that you know where you stand. One of the most common failures in the treatment of infertility is to allow the tests to drift on, often for years. This may result in a couple receiving inadequate or wrong treatment simply because the cause has not been correctly established. This can have tragic consequences, especially if the woman is in her late 30s and time is running out. A common problem is when one cause is found halfway through infertility testing; treatment is then immediately started without completing the rest of the tests. However, a couple may well have more than one problem contributing to their failure to conceive, and treatment of this without discovering the other one may prolong things unnecessarily.

Even experienced specialists (myself included) may occasionally forget to perform an important test. Although you may be in awe of your specialist (a totally illogical attitude in my view), you should certainly try to remind him or her if you feel that a special test might be helpful. This chapter provides you with a checklist. Many patients find it very difficult or embarrassing to be assertive. If you cannot summon up the courage to ask your specialist, talk things over with your family doctor. After all, he or she will have usually referred you to the specialist and is there to keep a watching brief over your general care. Tell your family doctor that you feel that certain tests are taking too long, or are not being done. A letter from him or her to the specialist, outlining your concerns, will frequently speed things up dramatically. You need not worry that the specialist will take offence. On the contrary, the specialist's practice depends on him or her satisfying the patients sent by family doctors.

What tests may be helpful before seeking specialist help?

In the early days of trying for a baby, three simple tests may help identify a problem. These can be organized by your family doctor, before referral to a specialist is considered.

- *Temperature charting.* A woman's temperature rises slightly after ovulation and remains raised until the next menstrual period. It may be worth taking your temperature for two or three months to see if you are ovulating. You should be aware that temperature charting is not very reliable (*see below* "The pitfalls of temperature charting") and that it has other disadvantages, such as causing unreasonable anxiety and tension.
- *The woman can have a blood test* to see if she is ovulating. The family doctor can easily arrange to have blood progesterone levels measured in the second half of the menstrual cycle. A well-raised level is excellent evidence of ovulation.
- *The man could have a simple sperm test.* This may show that there are inadequate numbers of normal sperm, in which case early specialist referral is justified.

Referral to a specialist or infertility clinic

If you don't conceive within two years, or if you are in any of the situations I have already described, your family doctor will refer you to a specialist. This will usually be a consultant, often a gynaecologist, who has an interest in infertility. If you have a clinic or specialist in mind and you would like to be specifically referred there, you are entitled to ask your family doctor. Many people worry about whether the woman should go on her own, or whether both partners should go to the specialist for the first visit. Generally, I think it is better if the couple attends together – for the first appointment, at least – as this means that you can share, and reduce, the tensions involved in visits to a specialized infertility clinic. Most specialists are pleased if both partners come.

What happens at a first appointment?

In the previous chapters, we looked at various symptoms. These lead to the main questions you might expect the doctor to ask. Obviously, age is important and the length of time a couple have been trying to have a baby. A history of any previous pregnancies is important and whether the woman found it difficult to conceive then. If the woman used to get pregnant easily, it suggests that something has happened to change her fertility.

Some women are very worried that they may be asked about a previous pregnancy (or abortion) about which their partners have no knowledge. If this is the case, it is best to be candid with your doctor, possibly waiting, for a time when you can talk to him on your own, perhaps at a subsequent clinic visit when you may want to come by yourself. He or she will not reveal this information to anybody else, including your present partner.

A gynaecological history will be needed, and it helps if the woman comes with the dates of recent menstrual periods. The specialist will also need to know about the frequency of sexual intercourse. A very few people still find these things embarrassing, but obviously how often you have sex is relevant. You need not be at all shy about these sorts of details. Every consultant gynaecologist is used to a very wide variety of problems and difficulties, and he or she certainly will not embarrass you at all with detailed questions.

Some women are naturally worried about a pelvic examination. If you find this especially embarrassing, you should certainly say so. In practice, provided a woman is having regular normal intercourse and there are no womb abnormalities or an ovarian cyst, remarkably little useful information is gained by an internal examination. This can also be deferred until a subsequent visit, when you have gained confidence. Examination of the man also often gives limited information, unless he has an abnormal sperm count. Even then, most men will be found to be completely normal on examination.

What tests are there for infertility?

Infertility tests can really be divided into three types: essential, optional, and the more or less useless. The first group, the "essential" tests, consist of those which can be done immediately after your first attendance at an infertility clinic or those which take time to organize but are generally essential in nearly all cases of infertility. The second group of "optional" tests are specialized and are not required in every case, but may be helpful if either (1) you do not get pregnant fairly soon (normally within six months) after treatment is started, or (2) if the cause of your infertility cannot be clearly established. There is also a third group of tests – which I term "useless". They may be done, but there is, in my opinion, very little rational basis for them.

No two specialists will do tests in precisely the same order. For example, many will prefer to do a laparoscopy before ordering a hysterosalpingogram. Others will substitute one kind of test for another. What I have done in this section is to try to lay out my own preferences, with the order of tests that generally make most sense in my own practice. Tests should be done in a logical fashion and without undue waiting so that they are completed within a reasonable length of time. They should also be explained to you and the results clearly given to you.

Essential tests for the man

Sperm count
Male problems are as likely as female ones, and sperm counts, or *semen analyses*, are essential. You should, however, remember three very important points. First, a single normal sperm count does not completely exclude a male problem. As we shall see, a man may

produce many sperm, freely moving around, but there are subtle problems with them which may prevent fertilization. Second, an abnormal or low count does not mean that there is necessarily something wrong. Most men produce poor-quality semen from time to time, especially if they are under stress. Good clinics always do several sperm counts before pronouncing on the male's fertility. Third, although a man may have previously fathered a pregnancy he may now be infertile. Men – like women – become infertile after various problems.

How is the sperm count done?

You, or your partner, will be given a little pot together with a form – usually asking you to fill in a few basic details. Semen needs to be delivered to the clinic within about 2 hours of its production. Most men prefer to produce it by masturbation; some like their partners to help them; and others find it easier to produce semen by interrupting intercourse, and ejaculating into the little pot. A good infertility clinic will give clear written instructions about the method of collection they prefer and how soon the semen is needed after collection for analysis. Some clinics prefer a couple not to have had intercourse for three days before a test, though opinions vary about how important this is.

Unfortunately, most clinics tend to give very small pots to men. Don't be embarrassed if you miss the pot, or if not all the semen gets in – just record this information on the form. Missing part of the semen may make the count abnormally low, but it always can be repeated at a later date. Do not use a condom for sperm collection: most contain substances which kill the sperm.

What is a "normal" sperm count?

The sperm will be sent to a laboratory where it will be examined under a microscope for the following qualities:

● *Semen volume*. Normally between 2–5ml (up to a teaspoonful). If low, the man may not be producing enough secretions. Alternatively, part of the sample may not have been collected at ejaculation. While a man may think that he is very virile if he is able to produce a large volume, much over 5 ml may dilute the sperm too much.

● *Sperm numbers*. Should be greater than 40 million in each millilitre. If below 20 million, you may have a problem. Some men, however, are fully fertile when they produce only 2 or 3 million sperm per millilitre of semen. Why this is so is not understood.

- *Sperm motility.* At least 40 per cent of the sperm should be moving under their own steam. If the motility is much below this, it is very likely there is a problem.
- *Normal sperm.* At least 65 per cent of the sperm should look normal under a microscope. If there are many abnormal sperm, there may be a serious problem with their manufacture in the testicles.
- *"Clumping" bacteria, white blood cells.* A good lab will also record whether there is any "clumping" (i.e. sperm stuck together). This may indicate an infection, or possibly antibodies to the sperm. If this is the case, specialized sperm tests are needed (*see below*). Many white cells or "debris", or obvious bacteria, may indicate an infection, making the sperm abnormal.
- *Chemical tests.* Some labs routinely test for certain chemicals such as fructose (*see* p. 121).
- *Antibodies.* Many laboratories routinely test for antibodies that may be attacking the sperm (*see* p. 120).

Getting your sperm count results

I strongly recommend that, when you return to your doctor to get the result of the sperm count, you both try to go together. The test result is emotionally very important to each of you for different reasons, and it can be a considerable burden for the woman to go on her own and find out that her man has a problem. Not surprisingly, most women do not want to be the one who has to break the news of a low sperm count. You should also not expect a good clinic to give these results to you over the telephone. For one thing, they can never be sure to whom they are speaking. For another, they cannot give you proper emotional support (if it is needed) over the telephone.

When getting the sperm count results, it is essential to bear in mind that perfectly fertile men may have an abnormal semen test from time to time. A single bad test result is simply not diagnostic on its own, so neither of you should be depressed or worried if the first count is below average, or even if there is no sperm present in the sample. This is surprisingly common.

The post-coital test

This is done after sexual intercourse (*coitus*), preferably some 6–36 hours later. The specialist simply takes a sample of fluid from the woman's cervix during a simple internal examination; this is similar to a cervical smear test. He or she then immediately examines the cervical fluid or mucus under a microscope and checks whether sperm are present, and whether the sperm are moving around. This test needs to be performed during the first half of the woman's menstrual cycle, just before ovulation when the mucus is most easily penetrated by the sperm.

Strictly speaking, the post-coital test is not only a test of the man's fertility, but also helps to show that ovulation may be occurring in the woman, that her cervix is healthy and that there is no obvious compatibility problem between the two of you.

It is a pity that this test is sometimes neglected as it gives very useful information, both about the quality of the sperm and about the cervical mucus.

The reasons for a negative post-coital test

The following reasons why a post-coital test result might be negative are listed in order of the most to the least common.

1. The test has been done too late in the woman's cycle, when ovulation has already occurred, after which cervical mucus production virtually dries up.

2. The test has been done too early in the woman's cycle, before oestrogen is produced in large enough amounts to influence mucus manufacture.

3. The test has been done during a cycle when the woman happens not to ovulate.

4. The man just produced poor semen this time.

5. Sperm are not being produced in sufficient quantity, or their quality is not really ideal.

6. The woman has a persistent problem with failure to ovulate.

7. The woman's cervix is abnormal and is therefore producing abnormal, impenetrable mucus.

8. The woman has a scarred or infected cervix which is not producing enough mucus.

9. Either of you is producing antibodies which are attacking the sperm.

10. The man is not ejaculating into the vagina properly.

Note that the first four reasons all occur in normal couples and are the most common reasons for a negative test.

Myths surrounding the post-coital test

● *A negative test is caused by a tilted (retroverted) uterus.* Wrong: 25 per cent of women have a uterus which is lying in a retroverted position. There is no real evidence that this influences the post-coital test or female fertility.

● *A negative test is caused by the sperm flowing out of the vagina after intercourse.* Wrong. All women, provided there is a reasonable quantity of ejaculate, tend to lose fluid from the vagina after intercourse. This is completely normal and perhaps one of the reasons why God ensured that men produce many millions of sperm each time they make love.

● *The test is negative because you are not having sex in the missionary position.* Wrong. There is no evidence at all that position during intercourse has the slightest influence on fertility. Indeed, I know from personal experience that a woman can conceive standing upright.

● *The post-coital test will be negative if it is not done within 2 or 3 hours of sexual intercourse.* Wrong. Despite the fact that even many doctors seem to believe this, a properly done test will be positive at least 8 hours after intercourse and usually much longer. If a proper search is made, it should be possible to identify active sperm 72 hours after having sex. This is important because too many clinics demand that the unfortunate woman must rush up to the hospital immediately after making love so that the test can be performed. This can throw a totally unnecessary strain on to both partners and many men become totally impotent when such unreasonable demands are made. If you are caught in this situation, you should certainly hold out for your rights.

● *A negative test means that the woman is killing off her partner's sperm.* Wrong. All couples frequently have negative post-coital tests; the test needs to be persistently negative before it can be said that there is any real likelihood that something is wrong.

Essential tests for the woman

Testing for ovulation

These tests should certainly be organized at the first visit. Good clinics employ more than one test for ovulation to confirm that the ovaries really are working.

Blood test for progesterone

This is the most important and most widely used test for ovulation. Actually, it only gives circumstantial evidence that ovulation has taken place, as it simply measures the amount of the hormone progesterone produced by the ovary – it does not detect whether an egg really left the ovary. As we have seen (*see* Chapter 1), progesterone is one of the female hormones produced by the ovary, mostly during the second half of the cycle.

There are two different ways of expressing these hormone measurements, either "nmol per litre" (common in Britain) or "ng per litre" (common in the US). The normal level following ovulation is 30 nmol per litre or 10 ng per litre depending on which measurement is used. If the progesterone in your blood level rises to these levels, it is almost certain that you are ovulating normally.

These levels are not reached immediately after ovulation, but about a week later and are maintained for three to five days. This is why it is usual to measure this hormone on the 21st day of your menstrual cycle, and why good clinics often repeat the blood test two or three days later to confirm that the rise is maintained. The level falls sharply immediately before your period, so a test taken within a day or two of bleeding may be meaningless. This is very important to understand, because many couples become discouraged when they have a low reading – this result may simply be because the first day of your period occurred earlier or later than expected.

One warning: If you are taking the fertility drug clomiphene (Clomid), any measurement of the blood progesterone level can be misleading. Because clomiphene increases the number and size of the follicles in the ovary as well as helping you to ovulate, you can produce a high level of progesterone even though you haven't actually ovulated. Unfortunately, many clinics (and, dare I say, doctors) forget this and patients can be lulled into a sense of false security. Therefore, if you are taking Clomid tablets, ultrasound tests are much more reliable (*see* p. 225).

Temperature charts

Temperature charting could actually be put into my third category of tests – those of little value. A great many books, and some clinics, seem to place great importance on temperature charting. Because it just might be helpful for a month or two when starting tests, here's how to do it.

Collect from your clinic, or buy from your chemist, a standard fertility temperature chart. Each morning, throughout your cycle, you should take your temperature with a clinical thermometer(which will show even slight variations in temperature), also available from some clinics or bought from the chemist. This should be done first thing on waking, before getting out of bed, drinking the cup of tea that your partner always brings you, or smoking a cigarette. Your temperature should be taken by placing the thermometer under your tongue for at least one minute. (Incidentally, the French, for reasons I have never understood, advise taking the temperature by inserting the thermometer into the rectum. There seems to be a popular belief, apparently held by some continental physicians, that things inserted rectally are more effective.) As soon as you have measured your temperature, you record this on your chart, which, of course, is always to hand on the bedside table.

The pitfalls of temperature charts While it is true that a woman's body temperature rises slightly after ovulation (probably because the increased levels of progesterone increase her metabolism), many perfectly normally ovulating women never have an appreciable change. If you are in this group and you are charting your temperature, you would be wrongly disappointed and distressed. On the other hand, some women who are not ovulating effectively do notice some rise in temperature after the mid-cycle, and if you are in this group, you may be being misled into thinking your ovaries are working properly.

Finally, but most important, some women are led to believe that their temperature chart will tell them when they are at their most fertile and use the chart to time intercourse. As we have already seen, the best time to conceive is by making love 12–48 hours before ovulation – this is, of course, before the temperature starts rising. It is true that, just before ovulation, some women experience an apparent fall in temperature; some "authorities" recommend using this to time sex. Unfortunately, there are a great many reasons why your temperature may fall and this is a most unreliable sign.

The objections to keeping a temperature chart
● They are generally very unreliable and can be misleading.
● They are a constant reminder that you are desperately trying to get pregnant.

● They can be infuriatingly inconvenient, especially if you are travelling or on holiday, or busy working, particularly if you are on night shifts.

● They encourage many couples to make love to order, destroying spontaneity. This, for my money, is the most important objection. You are convinced, from the drop in temperature this morning, that tonight's the night. Your husband comes home after a row with his boss, dog-tired. You forget to put the cat out, or burn the soup. He doesn't feel sexy. You end up half-trying to have intercourse, but certainly not making love. Both of you finish by feeling bad. This, a not untypical scenario, repeated in different ways each month, can be extremely demoralizing.

The advantages of temperature charting
● They give you a chance to do something which might help.
● They help you take some control of your problem away from the doctors and back to where it belongs, with you and your partner.
● They are quite a good way of keeping a record of your period dates – if you can stand it.
● For a few women, they are not inconvenient and are quite reliable.

If you do decide to do a temperature chart, I suggest that you set a time limit on the number of months for this experiment. You should also get supporting evidence of the chart's reliability in your case by alternative, simultaneous tests. Finally, do not attempt to time your sex life using a temperature chart.

Endometrial biopsy
An endometrial biopsy is a test in which a tiny piece of the uterine lining (*endometrium*) is examined under the microscope. Provided the biopsy is done during the second half of the menstrual cycle, it gives helpful information about ovulation. It tells whether or not the uterine lining has been exposed to and has responded to the progesterone that is normally produced by the ovary after ovulation.

How an endometrial biopsy is done   The best time is from the 19th day of a 28-day cycle up to the time of menstruation. The cervix is cleaned with soapy solution, after a simple examination. A small metal pipe is inserted through the opening of the cervix, and a tiny scraping of the lining of the uterus is removed within a few seconds, and placed in fixative on a slide to be later stained and examined in the laboratory. This procedure can cause brief discomfort – usually a little cramping like a period pain. Recently, various methods of taking a biopsy with a fine plastic sucker have been introduced, and this is more comfortable.

Because a few women do feel unhappy or frightened about the discomfort occasionally experienced during this test, it is very common for many clinics (my own included) to delay this test until the patient comes into hospital for laparoscopy under anaesthesia.

Testing the tubes and uterus
The hysterosalpingogram

The hysterosalpingogram (or HSG, for short) is an X-ray of the uterus and Fallopian tubes. Sadly, it is a rather neglected test and some doctors even believe that the need for it has been replaced by laparoscopy. In fact, a properly done HSG gives information impossible to get by other methods. During the test, a little dye is placed into the uterus and X-rays are taken. The tubes can be viewed to see whether they are open or not, but more importantly, the quality of the shadow on the X-ray can give very good detail of the outline of the inside of the uterus – very difficult to achieve by other methods – and the shadows produced by the tubes themselves give a good idea of not only tubal blockage but whether there is extensive scarring unsuitable for surgical treatment.

It is quite important that the specialist looks at the actual X-rays, rather than the report which comes from the radiologist. One patient of mine, who lived abroad came to see me with the following report:

Mrs S.S. X-ray of baby bag reveals creating of spray alright with no rocks. Egg basket poor visualized with good hatsatsora shadowed by agen; lulaot liquid observed in both trumpets but not captivated and query spilling but its not clear from which side. [I like "not clear from which side". Fortunately, the X-rays themselves were a bit more informative.]

When should a hysterosalpingogram be done? We organize an HSG to be done as soon as we can after a woman has first attended our clinic. This means that when the couple return for the first follow-up visit, we have valuable information about the quality of the woman's tubes and the inside of her uterus. There are certain situations, though, when the HSG may be better done after a laparoscopy – for example, if you know that you have some form of tubal damage.

It is unwise to have any X-ray of the abdomen if there is even the slightest possibility that you might be pregnant. Because of this, it is best for the HSG to be performed during the first half of the cycle, before ovulation. If you are attending a busy hospital, and it is difficult to get an appointment for an HSG in the first two weeks of your cycle, it is perfectly all right to have the X-ray more than two weeks after your period, provided you use some effective contraception (say, a condom) during that month. The HSG should not be done during the period itself, because it is thought that this may be a cause of endometriosis.

What should you expect?   On the day of your appointment, you go to the X-ray department. Following a simple internal examination on the X-ray couch, the doctor inserts a small tube through the opening of the cervix. This tube is thin – the part which actually fits inside the cervix is no larger than a ball-point pen refill. Fitting this may cause fleeting discomfort – certainly no worse than that experienced with a period. A small amount of dye is gently injected into the uterus, and the progress of the dye can be seen on a television screen and X-rays can be taken. Usually about six of these are taken, and the procedure takes 10 minutes. This procedure does not require hospital admission or an anaesthetic and is painless in most cases.

While it is true that the HSG has a bad reputation for causing discomfort, this is now quite unjustified. If modern techniques are used (especially the newer, less irritant X-ray dyes) and the doctor is gentle and the dye injected slowly, most women do not realize the test has started or finished. However, because many are nervous about the test and a very few do have crampy discomfort, it is sensible to be accompanied at your X-ray appointment by your partner or a friend. They can give you moral support and a bit of company on the way home if you feel a bit sore. Persistent pain after the HSG (particularly hours later) is definitely abnormal. If you experience this, you should phone the hospital, no matter how late at night, for advice.

What information does a hysterosalpingogram give which other tests do not?   Laparoscopy is just as good, if not better, at telling whether the tubes are open. Nevertheless, HSG gives unique information about:

114

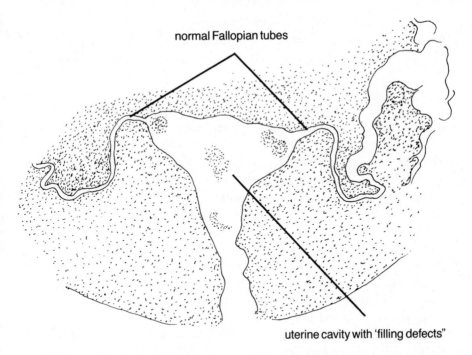

normal Fallopian tubes

uterine cavity with 'filling defects"

Hysterosalpingogram (HSG). Special X-ray dye has been injected through the cervix (at the bottom of the picture), and the inside of the uterine cavity and Fallopian tubes are outlined by the dye. In this woman the tubes are normal and open, but there are areas in the uterine cavity that have not filled — possibly due to fibroids.

● *The inside of the uterus.* It is very good at showing adhesions inside the womb, as well as fibroids, adenomyosis and polyps.

● *The area where the tubes join the uterus.* This area, the internal plumbing which is exceptionally delicate and small, is poorly seen at laparoscopy. The HSG gives an idea whether there is any scar tissue in this area, or polyps in the tube itself.

● *The lining of the tube.* The tubal lining and its folds show up very nicely on a well-taken X-ray. This helps to decide if your tubes are scarred.

● *How scarred the tubes are,* if they are blocked. This gives important information about whether surgery is worth considering.

Unfortunately what the HSG cannot give information about (though this is sometimes claimed) are adhesions around the Fallopian tubes, endometriosis or scarring of the abdominal lining.

Laparoscopy

This is the most informative and important test for female infertility. If I was on a desert island (equipped with a modern operating theatre, of course) and allowed only one test for infertility, this would be it. It involves inserting a thin telescope into the abdominal cavity through a small hole made in the navel. In order to get a good view, a little carbon dioxide gas is first passed into the cavity. This separates all the organs and makes their anatomy easy to identify. The telescope is no thicker than a fountain pen, but due to the remarkable development of modern optics, the view obtained is superb. Moreover, photographs of very high quality can be taken via the telescope – a facility which more and more surgeons are using. Through the laparoscope, the surgeon can inspect your uterus, test your tubes to see if they are open or scarred on the outside, and look at your ovaries. It is true to say that laparoscopy – far more than test-tube baby treatment or any other development – has been the single most revolutionary advance in infertility diagnosis and treatment.

When is laparoscopy indicated?   I think that laparoscopy is useful in any woman who has been trying to get pregnant for longer than two years. It is indicated earlier if there is any reason to suspect a tubal problem, or in older women when time is running out. It is also vital if you have previously had any abdominal or gynaecological surgery.

What does a laparoscopy involve?   In general, it is best done in the second half of your cycle, so that the surgeon can examine your ovaries to see if ovulation has happened.

Although a few surgeons have experimented with laparoscopy under local anaesthesia, a general anaesthetic with the patient asleep is now far more common. Laparoscopy requires admission to hospital, usually overnight. A few centres now do laparoscopy as a day-care procedure, usually to cut costs. If you are having laparoscopy on this basis, without staying overnight, you will normally be expected to arrive at the hospital or clinic by about 8.00 o'clock in the morning, ready for a light general anaesthetic. You should have not eaten or drunk anything since midnight because having anaesthesia

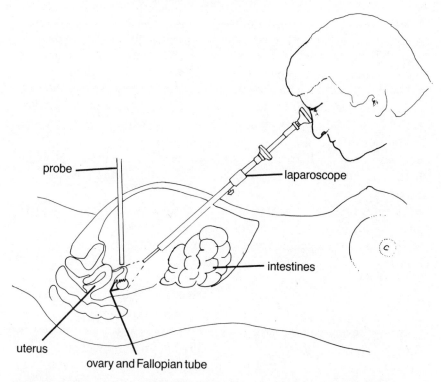

probe

laparoscope

intestines

uterus

ovary and Fallopian tube

Laparoscopy. Carbon dioxide gas has already been injected into the tummy to separate the organs so that the surgeon gets a good view down the telescope.

with any food or drink in your stomach is unsafe. If you have been recently unwell, or if you have a heavy head-cold, for example, you should inform the hospital, who may wish you to postpone your laparoscopy until you are completely fit.

The procedure itself takes from between 10–40 minutes and carries no serious risk to you. When you wake up afterwards you will normally find two small dressings on your tummy. One will cover a single stitch in your navel, the other a tiny hole near the pubic hairline. This second hole is used to place any fine probes in your abdominal cavity which may be required to get a better view. Most people have very little discomfort and no pain after laparoscopy; others may feel a bit sore. A very few women do feel distinctly unwell and need to rest in bed for 24 hours. The commonest side-effects are:

- Soreness in the tummy (usually not at all bad).

117

● Soreness or pain in one or other shoulder. This may seem a strange place to feel discomfort. It is due to irritation from the carbon dioxide gas which stimulates the nerves to your abdominal lining. These are the same nerves that supply the shoulder area, hence the discomfort.

● Vaginal bleeding. This may occur because the surgeon has manipulated the cervix during the injection of the dye to check the tubes. The bleeding is usually heavy enough to warrant wearing a sanitary towel for two or three days, and it may go on longer.

● A sore throat. This may occur because the anaesthetist placed a breathing tube down your throat to ensure a safe anaesthetic. This soreness rarely lasts longer than 24 hours.

● Sleeplessness the night after or vivid dreams. This is a frequent effect of any procedure involving general anaesthesia.

● Sickness. Some people feel sick after having an anaesthetic. Fewer do these days because the action of the drugs is so much gentler than in times past. If you are prone to sickness after anaesthesia, you should tell the anaesthetist or nurses beforehand as they can usually give you special drugs which reduce this unpleasant problem.

If you have laparoscopy done on a daycare basis, you will rest in hospital for 4–6 hours afterwards. Following this, you will be allowed home; because you may feel a bit dizzy, you need to be accompanied by someone. You should avoid wetting the areas covered by the dressings for 48 hours. Most surgeons put an absorbable stitch in the navel and this will usually dissolve after two to four weeks, which saves you a hospital visit to have it removed.

What can be gained from laparoscopy?

● It is the best way of determining whether your tubes are damaged or blocked.

● It is extremely valuable in seeing if you have any adhesions in your abdominal cavity (*see* p. 91).

● It gives a direct view of the ovaries and, provided the laparoscopy is done in the second half of your cycle, the surgeon can see whether you have recently ovulated.

● It is the best way to detect endometriosis.

● It gives an excellent view of the outside of the uterus and may help to detect fibroids or a congenital problem in the womb.

● It is a useful aid to see if there are other diseases affecting your ovaries, such as cysts, or other diseases in the abdominal cavity.

● There is some evidence that, after laparoscopy, rather more women immediately conceive than would be expected by chance. About 15 per cent of our patients whose tubes are open conceive within three months of laparoscopy. The reason for this is not clear but may be due to the action of flushing the tubes with dye.

Optional tests for the man

The following tests may be helpful if your partner has more than one sperm count which is abnormal or low.

Separation test (swim test)
This also tests sperm function. Available in specialist centres, it involves placing the semen in special fluids to see how many sperm can swim properly. The normal sperm separate from the abnormal ones, giving an idea of how many may be capable of fertilizing an egg. Those of us in our unit think that this is a really worthwhile test.

One of the problems with this test is that the semen needs to be quite fresh. Most clinics like the semen to be produced in the hospital, but few hospitals offer really adequate facilities for producing semen, and most men have to produce semen in the nearest lavatory. In some hospitals, a proper bedroom is available; very often this is oversubscribed, resulting in the embarrassment of the men queuing up to use the "facilities". If ever a man needs a sense of humour and perspective during infertility tests, now is the time.

Computer sperm motility tests
An increasing number of laboratories are using computerized measurement of sperm function and motility. Sperm are observed under a microscope to which a television camera is attached; their movements are digitized by a computer – usually an IBM with extra memory chips – and then the quality of the movement of individual sperm is assessed. This may be helpful in assessing how "good" the sperm are. This test is more widely available in the United States than in Britain, partly because of the technological enthusiasm there and partly because of financial reasons. However, there is no good evidence that digitized computer sperm counting is much of an improvement over simpler methods.

Hormone tests
A very few men with low sperm counts have a hormonal problem.

Occasionally, the pituitary gland may not be producing enough LH or FSH (the same hormones that regulate a woman's menstrual cycle), and this is measurable and treatable. Conversely, high levels of these hormones suggest that no treatment is likely to be of assistance. Measurement of the male hormone *testosterone* may also help decide whether the testicles are capable of working normally. Sometimes the hormone *prolactin* is also measured. Produced by the pituitary gland in both men and women, in women it stimulates the production of breast milk. In rare cases, it may be abnormally high in men; however, this test is of dubious value.

Testicular biopsy

This is done by a surgeon who removes a tiny sliver of tissue from a testicle and "fixes" it in a special solution. It is also usual to examine the epididymis (the tube close to the testicle) at the same time to see if it looks diseased or blocked. The procedure requires an anaesthetic and an overnight hospital stay. Microscopic examination of the tissue sample will reveal whether the testis is producing sperm or not. If it is not producing sperm properly, you may have to face the fact that there is no real treatment. Testicular biopsy is really only worth doing in a small percentage of cases.

Testicular X-rays (vasography)

This may be done at the time of a testicular biopsy. A little dye is squirted into the vas deferens. This may establish whether or not there is a blockage which may be worth operating upon. These X-rays are excessively pretty – if you have this done, be sure to ask to have a look.

Thermography

This is used in some centres, mostly in the United States, to assess the temperature of the testicles. The man places his testicles over a heat-sensitive plate, which then changes colour (like the paper thermometers bought in chemists' shops). If the plate turns blue, this means that one of the testicles is hot and that there may be a varicocoele present (*see* p. 132). I am not convinced that this test, nor testicular ultrasound, is particularly useful. Thermography is at least totally painless, and the pretty colours are fun.

Antibody testing

Some men certainly produce antibodies which identify the sperm (or parts of them – such as the heads or the tails) as foreign protein. This results in the sperm sticking together, or being deficient in other ways – particularly in being less able to propel themselves around. Two tests may be done to detect antibodies: the MAR test, done on the semen, the Kibrick test, done on blood. Unless the levels of antibody are clearly high, there is considerable doubt about the relevance of these tests. Sperm clumping can also be caused by infection.

Sperm culture

If an infection is suspected, some laboratories culture the semen to try to identify the bacterium responsible before antibiotic treatment is undertaken. These cultures tend to be quite unreliable, which is why they are by no means done routinely.

Fructose measurement

If there are no sperm in the semen, there may be a blockage either above or below the seminal vesicles. The seminal vesicles produce fructose, a simple sugar which is easily measured in semen. If the semen is low in fructose, this suggests that the blockage is below the seminal vesicles, which helps direct a surgeon where to look.

Split ejaculate test

During ejaculation, it is usual for the first part of the semen to be richer in sperm, even when the sperm count is a bit low. This "concentrated" semen may be worth collecting for subsequent artificial insemination (*see* Chapter 11). The split ejaculate test helps evaluate this. It is devillishly hard to do, as it involves the man juggling between two collecting pots – usually while masturbating. Even performers at the Moscow State Circus would find this difficult. Sometimes a partner can be very helpful here. Infertility treatment is sometimes a remarkable way of overcoming life's little sensitivities.

Hamster test

This involves testing the sperm to see if they are capable of penetrating the eggs of a golden hamster. A simple sperm count does not always give a good idea about whether the sperm actually function normally. One theoretical way of getting around this problem is to see how they react in contact with eggs from other mammals. It has been found that the hamster egg is a reasonably good model. The prepared semen are mixed with the hamster eggs and the number of eggs which are penetrated by sperm is counted. (Rest assured that a hamster egg penetrated by human sperm is completely incapable of developing into an embryo.) If no eggs are penetrated, this suggests that the sperm function is inadequate in some way. Recent evidence suggests that this test is not very reliable and so it has been largely abandoned – quite good news for hamsters.

Karyotype (chromosome) test

For this, the blood is usually tested. Some men who produce very few or no sperm have a genetic (chromosomal) problem. A chromosome count can reveal this. Unfortunately, there is no treatment if this is the problem.

The human zona penetration test

The ability of a sperm to penetrate the zona (the "shell") of the egg is an important function. To test this, the sperm can be mixed with dead human eggs obtained from a "spare" ovary removed during hysterectomy. Even if the sperm penetrate the outer layer, there in no risk of an embryo being formed as the egg itself is dead. It is presently available only in research centres.

In vitro fertilization (IVF)

"Washed" sperm can be mixed with a live egg taken from an ovary just before ovulation. This is, in fact, an extension of the test-tube baby process. If an embryo develops, this is, of course, the best proof that the sperm are capable of normal activity. Any embryo that is obtained can be put back into the woman's uterus, where it may develop into a baby. In many ways, this is the ultimate test of sperm function; the reason why it is not done more often is because it is very expensive. It is, of course, available only at some centres where IVF is done.

An optional test for both partners: Crossed mucus penetration test (mucus hostility test)

This may be used when the man's sperm count is more or less

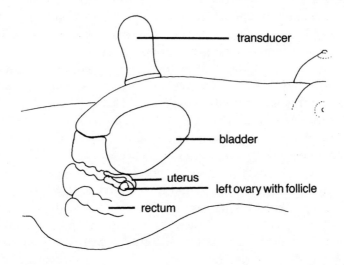

Ultrasound examination. The sound waves are sent from the transducer to structures in the abdominal cavity, where they bounce back to the transducer again. These reflections are then translated into a picture on a TV screen.

normal, but the post-coital test is repeatedly negative. It involves examining under a microscope either a sample of the man's sperm combined with cervical mucus from a donor, or donor sperm mixed with the woman's mucus. This may help decide whether it is the male or female partner who is producing antibodies that are killing off the sperm.

Optional tests for the woman

These tests are done by an increasing number of clinics, particularly if the cause of infertility is unclear, or if a subtle problem with ovulation is suspected.

Ovarian ultrasound

This is very useful – so useful that many specialists try it first. Ultrasonic sound waves are aimed at the ovaries through the abdominal wall, and the echoes obtained can be picked up and displayed on a television screen. It is very similar to the sonar used on ships. Modern ultrasound allows very precise measurement (to the nearest milli-metre) of many structures inside your abdomen. Ultrasound works best through water, which is an excellent conductor of sound. This is why abdominal ultrasound is performed when you have a really full bladder – it gives a better picture of the ovaries, which lie just behind the bladder. Some well-equipped clinics also have vaginal ultrasound – a small ultrasound probe can be put in the vagina and an excellent view of the ovaries obtained. This has many advantages for you – filling the bladder full enough for abdominal ultrasound can be very, uncomfortable.

The ultrasound helps to decide whether or not the follicles in your ovaries are growing normally, and it can also detect when they have just ruptured, that is, when you have ovulated. Usually this rupture should happen when the follicles are about 18–22 millimetres in diameter. Ultrasound is also very helpful in identifying whether you have polycystic ovaries (*see* p. 83). It is also an excellent way of detecting an early pregnancy.

Hormone profiles
Some clinics find it helpful to measure the levels of hormones in your blood or urine on a more or less daily basis for the best part of an entire menstrual cycle. This may help pinpoint a subtle abnormality in your hormones, which may be responsible for your failure to ovu-late properly. It is customary to measure the hormones oestrogen, LH and progesterone, and compare the results with the levels of a group of women known to be ovulating normally.

Measurement of LH and FSH
This is often useful if there is an ovulatory problem. If the levels of these two hormones is low, you may need to be given pituitary hor-mones. If the levels are a little raised, your ovaries may be polycystic. Rarely, LH and FSH may be very high indeed; unfortunately, this suggests that the ovaries may not have any eggs in them and that you are likely to be in a menopausal state.

Testosterone measurement
Raised levels of male hormone (which women also produce norm-ally) suggests that you may not be ovulating. This may be seen with certain types of polycystic ovary syndrome. It can also, very rarely, be associated with other diseases of the ovaries or the adrenal glands.

Prolactin measurement

This hormone is frequently raised, but infrequently causes a problem. Unfortunately, many women become very alarmed when told they have a high prolactin level. It is worth remembering that if your *progesterone* level is normal and consistent with that needed for ovulation to occur, a raised prolactin level is irrelevant. A high prolactin level only needs treating (with drugs, usually) if you are definitely not ovulating.

Skull X-ray and eye test

If your prolactin is raised, this may be because you have an enlarged pituitary gland which is overactive but not producing LH or FSH. Very rarely, this swelling can be a benign tumour. An X-ray of the skull in the region of the pituitary gland may detect such a problem. Because your visual fields (how far around you can see) can be affected, the doctor may want to test your eyes as well.

Thyroid hormone measurement

Very frequently measured, this is very infrequently the cause of failure to ovulate. Thyroid problems cause less than 1 per cent of infertility due to ovulation failure in most clinics.

Karyotype (chromosome) test

Just as men with a chromosomal abnormality may not produce normal sperm, so might women not produce normal eggs if they have a similar problem. The blood can be tested, and the result usually takes at least three to four weeks. These abnormalities are rare.

Extra tests for the tubes or uterus

These may occasionally be helpful, but many centres do not have facilities for them.

Hysteroscopy

This test involves passing a small telescope – called an *hysteroscope* – into the uterus. It is usually done under quick general anaesthetic, and you only have to come in for the day. It is valuable to see the inside of the uterus. Hysteroscopy is excellent at detecting any abnormalities that have been suspected after an HSG, such as polyps, uterine fibroids, a congenital abnormality or any adhesions which may scar the lining of the uterus. The hysteroscope can also be used to treat some of these conditions, by guiding fine scissors or other instruments inside the uterus.

Tuboscopy

A few specialists may wish to examine the inside of the Fallopian tubes, using a fine telescope. This is usually inserted through the abdomen wall while you are under general anaesthetic. It is a helpful but, as yet, not widely available technique, which aids in diagnosing areas of scarring or fine adhesions inside the tubes.

Tests of dubious value

Tubal insufflation

My own pet aversion is tubal insufflation. Regrettably, some patients are still offered this, and I would suggest that you firmly refuse. This test involves injecting carbon dioxide gas under pressure into the uterus. If the pressure does not rise above a certain level or the doctor can hear the gas bubbling through with a stethoscope or the unfortunate woman experiences pain in the tip of her shoulder, this is taken as evidence that gas is getting through the uterus and tubes. This may mean that the tubes are open.

This test is a museum piece. When it was invented – in 1919 by Dr Rubin of New York – it was reasonable because there was nothing better. It is painful, somewhat dangerous and very unreliable. The apparatus used to perform it is very beautiful to look at and would be best housed in a locked glass case in a mahogany cabinet.

D & C (dilatation & curettage)

Some women are still brought into hospital for a "womb scrape" if they are having difficulty in conceiving. Though harmless, it is valueless unless done at the time of a laparoscopy, when an endometrial biopsy is taken. It is performed because of a myth which suggests that it is easier to conceive after a D & C. There is no truth in this.

CHAPTER NINE

Routine Infertility Treatments

In Chapter 2, we looked at simple ways of helping yourself to get pregnant. We also saw the limitations of "self-help". Here we look at the various medical treatments available, what they have to offer, what they involve, and what kind of success rates may be expected. While obviously, as a doctor, I am biased in favour of active medical treatment, I have to say that all infertility treatment is limited. There are a few points worth remembering:

● Medical treatment is all very well, but many couples find it a huge help to feel that they have some control over the process.

● Many infertile couples achieve a pregnancy while undergoing no active treatment. Very few women, and only a few men, are ever completely sterile (even if treatment has failed).

● All active treatments for infertility are limited in success. Statistics from infertility clinics (including centres doing test-tube baby treatment) clearly show that *only 35 per cent of patients conceive as a result of the treatment they undergo.*

● It is, therefore, impossible for your doctor to predict the result of treatment. There are two things that few candid or truthful doctors can ever say to you: (1) "There is no chance of you conceiving" and (2) "This treatment will almost certainly help you have a baby."

Treatment for the man

There is no doubt that male infertility is very difficult to treat. All methods for improving sperm counts are extremely unreliable.

Worse still, if the sperm quality is poor, treatment to improve it may be totally useless. The basic problem is that we still do not understand why some sperm are healthy and others are not.

One of the greatest difficulties is that there is a peculiar paradox. If sperm are being produced at all, however few, there is always the possibility of success. Only one sperm is needed to produce a baby. This means that sometimes men with an apparently hopelessly low sperm count may eventually get their partners pregnant.

To add to the difficulties of prediction, some men produce very poor sperm for some years and then, quite suddenly and often without reason, start to produce much better quality sperm. Very frequently, if they are under treatment at the time, the improvement in sperm count is gratefully attributed to the therapy being given, but this may not be the true reason.

Even though simple remedies are unlikely to influence the complex events that contribute to sperm function, there is some real hope. Various measures are undoubtedly of value in improving male fertility, and some of them work quite dramatically.

General health measures

There is moderately good evidence that an improvement in general health may make a difference to male infertility. Many fertile men are prone to poor sperm counts, which may make them at least temporarily infertile. If the sperm count is marginal or low, certain health rules may maximize the chances of a baby. For example, the hazards described on pages 99–100 are relatively simple to correct, and this can be much more effective than other treatments with drugs. Perseverance with the suggestions recommended here is undoubtedly quite valuable, but remember that it takes about 70 days to make a sperm so the sperm count may not actually improve much for the first four months or so.

Lose excess weight

Losing excessive body weight by going on a suitable diet can be helpful. It is better to reduce gradually, losing around 2 lb (1 kilogram) each week. Crash dieting should be avoided.

Stop smoking

There can be no doubt that any smoking is bad for fertility. Anyone with a poor sperm count who smokes more than eight or ten cigarettes a day may well make any other fertility treatment useless. I try hard to encourage all my IVF patients to give up. If you have been a heavy smoker, you cannot expect your sperm count to return to normal levels immediately you give up the habit. It usually takes at least three months for any improvement to be clearly apparent.

Richard, a 33-year-old salesman, and his wife Jean came to see me after they had failed to have a baby after 11 years. She ovulated rather poorly and had been taking fertility drugs for seven years without a pregnancy. His sperm counts were always low, and artificial insemination had been tried many times without success. We measured his count four times in four successive months. The number of sperm per millilitre varied between 4 million and 9 million, the sperm's motility was never more than 30 per cent and usually about 40 per cent of the sperm showed some microscopic abnormality. I advised Richard to lose 20 lb (9 kilograms) and to stop smoking – at that time he was smoking 35–40 cigarettes a day. His work involved driving a great deal, but he didn't feel he could alter this much.

I saw him three months later. He had cut down to four cigarettes a day and had lost over 14 lb (6 kilograms). He continued with his normal work but was now exercising twice weekly – the first time in years. His sperm count on the day of his appointment was 56 million per millilitre and 50 per cent of the sperm were moving normally although about 30 per cent still showed some abnormality in shape. His sperm count remained at this level two months later. Five weeks after the second of these counts, his wife had a positive pregnancy test, and at the time of writing, Jean is in her second pregnancy!

Keep alcohol to a minimum

With everyone having a different physical reaction to drink, it is impossible to lay down the precise limits. The following would seem to be absolute maximum permitted amounts. A man with a depressed sperm count shouldn't drink more than 2–3 pints (1.5 litres) of beer daily. It follows that more than half a bottle of wine a day may be harmful. However, I have it on good authority that if the wine is from Burgundy and bottled by a good shipper, it may have a tonic effect. Spirits are thought to be particularly harmful, and two or three measures a day are enough.

Drugs

Medically prescribed drugs need to be discussed with your doctor. Obviously, drugs that are important to health cannot be stopped, but a change or a different dosage might be helpful.

Avoid excessive exercise

Regular marathon running or daily vigorous games of squash may be unwise. When physical training is taken too far, it is sensible to ease off for a while to see if the sperm count improves. One friend of mine, a regular marathon runner, found it very difficult to cut down on the amount of exercise he was doing even though his sperm counts were persistently low. However, within a few weeks of reducing the amount of exercise he did by half, the sperm count returned to virtually normal values – and his wife became pregnant three weeks later.

Reducing testicular temperature

Men are frequently told to take cold baths and wear loose-fitting underwear. There is very limited logic behind these suggestions. The testicles hang outside the body in the scrotum. This may possibly be nature's way of keeping them cooler than body temperature. It seems that sperm production is best when the testicles are several degrees cooler than 98.4° F (37°C) and it is just possible that close-fitting underwear, such as Y-fronts, cause overheating. Because of this, some doctors recommend men with low sperm counts to wear loose boxer shorts and even bathe the scrotum daily in very cold water. There is really no proof that any of this will help, and some couples feel it adds an element of torture to what is already an unpleasant situation. On the other hand, it does no harm and may be worth a go if only because it means that you are doing everything possible. Wearing loose-fitting underwear makes reasonable sense, and it seems a good idea to avoid very hot baths and saunas. You may be interested to know that, in some parts of the world (especially Japan), hot baths have been used as a method of male contraception. I would avoid cold water-treatments, however, as I am very unconvinced that they can be of real help.

Drug treatments

In my view, drug treatment is extremely limited in value. I think that many drugs are given largely because patients expect them and because it is much easier for the doctor to give some treatment rather than to be brutally frank. At least 200 different drugs have been prescribed over the years to improve sperm quality and numbers. That number says it all because, if there were a proven drug, there would have been far less "blunderbuss" treatment. The truth is that, except in a few specific cases, drugs are not likely to make much difference. This is, of course, depressing news, but it is important to recognize the problem from the outset. This will avoid your wasting a lot of time by taking different but equally ineffective drugs. It also will allow you to take proper decisions about what you should both do about the infertility.

The following are the drugs which are frequently tried.

Testosterone (male hormone)
Large doses of testosterone actually reduce the sperm count, so there is no point in long-term testosterone treatment. Some men, though, have a "rebound" effect. A short course of treatment with large doses of testosterone (given usually by injection) temporarily suppresses their sperm production When the drug is stopped, the testicles may "rebound" and there are claims that as many as 50 per cent of men will have a marked improvement in sperm count, though this effect will last only a short time.

Mesterolone (Pro-Viron)
This is a synthetic by-product of testosterone and is claimed to improve sperm motility and possibly sperm number. It is probably the most widely used drug for male infertility, but there is disappointingly little hard evidence that it improves fertility. We have used this drug extensively for very many years on large numbers of men; although some have shown improvements in sperm count, it is quite possible that this improved by itself. Very few of the men taking mesterolone have got their partners pregnant, probably no more than would have done so by chance.

Gonadotrophins (pituitary hormones FSH and LH)
These may be given by injection (Pergonal). Alternatively, LH may be given alone, usually as HCG (human chorionic gonadotrophin; brand names Pregnyl, Profasi). Claims have been made that, because these compounds increase the activity of the testicles, sperm counts may improve, rather than motility. In any case, their effect seems variable. They have been proved effective only for men with a pituitary abnormality, when normal production of FSH is decreased. These drugs are extremely expensive and treatment is lengthy; my feeling is that they are not justified unless there is a definite and well-defined hormone problem.

131

Clomiphene (Clomid) and tamoxifen (Tamotfen)

These are mostly used to stimulate the pituitary in women (*see below*); they also affect the ovary and uterus directly – sometimes unfavourably. They have occasionally been used to raise testosterone production by the testicles in the hope of improving the sperm count. Success has been very variable. We have used clomiphene and tamoxifen a lot in the past but have never been convinced that anyone we have given them to has benefited. We have now almost abandoned using this group of drugs for male infertility.

Antibiotics

There is little doubt that if you have an infection impairing sperm motility or quality, the chance of fertilization is reduced. Taking antibiotics may solve this problem as sperm motility often improves when any infection in the male genital tract is effectively treated. Treatment is usually needed for four to six weeks.

Immune therapy with steroids

If sperm counts are poor because of antibodies to the sperm, drugs may just be helpful. Corticosteroids are most commonly used, either prednisolone or ACTH. These drugs may be taken intermittently for several months and in quite high doses, and can be effective only if the testicles are not irreversibly damaged. They are not without quite serious side-effects, including stomach bleeding, mental depression, weight gain and a general feeling of being unwell. The usual practice is to give high doses of prednisolone for seven days or so each month to coincide with the woman's fertile period; such quick "in-and-out" treatment doesn't usually give time for any side-effects to develop. Whatever the situation, you should not take steroids for more than three or four months. It is claimed that about half of all men with antibodies may be helped by these drugs – that is, about 3 or 4 per cent of all infertile men.

You can also have the sperm "washed" in specially prepared solutions. The "washed" sperm can then be inseminated into the cervix with a little syringe. So far, this has had only limited success.

Surgery

Removing a varicocoele

Surgical correction of a varicose varicocoele, or vein in a testicle is very simple but there are conflicting opinions about its value. The problem is that about 20 per cent of both fertile and infertile men have a varicocoele and this seems no disadvantage to a fertile man. It is, however, thought that there is more chance of infertility if there is abnormal bloodflow in these varicose veins.

The operation involves tying off the abnormal vessels (ligation) or blocking them, usually with a chemical injection. If the injection method is used, a local anaesthetic is generally all that is needed. The procedure is neither painful nor dangerous and requires at most no more than one night in hospital. X-rays may be taken during surgery to confirm that the veins are effectively blocked. Some surgeons claim that at least 70 per cent of treated men will show an improvement in sperm count within three months. Others are less optimistic and some have not found that ligation of a varicocoele produces any improvement. Varicocoeles are usually quite painless and seldom even tender. They do not interfere with sex unless you knock them very hard indeed in a moment of great passion.

Unblocking the tubing

The tubes that carry sperm are very tiny. For example, the epididymis has an inner diameter of less than 0.2 millimetre – that is, the thickness of a piece of very fine cotton thread. The vas deferens is much thicker externally but it too is very narrow internally. If a blocked portion has to be removed and the tubing rejoined, the best results are obtained by microsurgery, with stitches so fine that they can hardly be seen at all with the naked eye. Although the surgery is technically difficult and a general anaesthetic is needed, recovery is very quick and there is hardly any pain so intercourse is not affected. A typical hospital stay is 2–4 days.

Results of microsurgery vary, depending on the position and extent of the block, and the expertise of the surgeon. If the tubing has been blocked for a long time, the testicle tends gradually to stop producing sperm. Unfortunately, if production stops altogether, more sperm may not be made even when the tubing is unblocked. Eight per cent of infertile men have a block, and 20 to 30 per cent will produce normal sperm after this type of operation.

Artificial insemination with the male partner's semen.

Artificial insemination is the technique whereby sperm are injected into the woman by artificial means. It is most frequently performed using sperm from a donor – and this is discussed in detail in the next

chapter. However, insemination with the male partner's semen –
commonly known as "artificial insemination by husband" (AIH)
may be recommended in some cases when the sperm count is poor.
Sperm can be inseminated by one of three well-tried methods.

Insemination into the cervix

Semen (usually produced by masturbation) is injected directly into
the vagina through a small plastic tube so that they reach the cervix.
The woman has to lie on a couch with her knees up for about five
minutes; the insemination itself causes no discomfort.

This kind of insemination is used for couples having difficulties
with sexual intercourse; it may also be useful in the rare event of
there being an anatomical problem with the uterus or cervix which
prevents sperm finding the right place. Although this is controversial,
I feel that there is usually little point in doing this if the man has a low
sperm count because natural intercourse will achieve the same end –
that is, introduction of sperm into the cervical canal. Although insemination causes no physical discomfort, the emotional pain may be
considerable. One theoretical advantage of AIH is that insemination
can be made at the most fertile moment – just before ovulation.

Using sperm that has been specially processed

The sperm are prepared after being produced by masturbation. They
may be "washed" – that is, the semen is repeatedly mixed with
special laboratory fluid, i.e. medium, and are then removed by centri-
fugal force, by spinning the tube containing them. Alternatively, the
sperm may be subjected to the "swim" test (*see* p. 119). The semen is
mixed with medium, healthy sperm are allowed to swim up to the
surface under their own steam and these are drawn off by suction
through a glass tube. These healthy, concentrated sperm may then be
inseminated into the cervix.

These methods may be used if there are large numbers of dead
sperm or many dead cells in the semen. Strictly speaking, no real con-
centration of semen takes place, just a purification. These methods
may also be used if there are sperm antibodies present, as the washing
process may get rid of these.

Another method of preparing semen involves using a split ejaculate
(*see* p. 121), to obtain the greater number of sperm that are present in
the first part of the ejaculate. These would then be inseminated into
the cervix.

When used appropriately, these methods can result in pregnancy in around 30 per cent of subfertile couples, provided that the couple is prepared to persevere with several cycles of treatment.

Intrauterine insemination

Occasionally doctors advise insemination directly into the uterus itself, bypassing the cervix. This is usually done when the woman has a cervical problem (*see* Chapter 6), but it is now being used for some cases of male infertility, especially when the sperm count is poor.

A fine tube containing sperm is inserted through the cervix and just into the uterus. This can cause minor discomfort, but there should be no pain. Fresh, unwashed semen cannot be used because of a risk of infection and the sperm need to be prepared in the laboratory. Early results are somewhat encouraging – a few doctors have had success with up to 40 per cent of couples.

Are there disadvantages to insemination with the male partner's sperm?

The disadvantages are so great that I would advise couples to agree to this treatment for only a limited time – say, no more than six months at most. The disadvantages include the following:

● The process itself tends to be very clinical and unspontaneous, and for some people, this is almost worse than being infertile. There is no doubt that this treatment invades your sex life to a greater extent than most doctors are prepared to admit or even realize.

● The man may not be able to masturbate to order. At the least, this will be embarrassing and, at worst, will cause feelings of guilt, frustration and anger. A great deal of patience and understanding are needed by both partners.

● Reasonably precise timing of ovulation is necessary. Temperature charting is insufficient, and your clinic should ask you to go in for blood tests, ultrasound or both. Regrettably, far too many clinics do not time this demanding treatment properly, so any benefit may be lost.

● Collecting a split ejaculate requires considerable manual dexterity right at the moment of orgasm.

● Sperm washing and the swim-up method require advanced laboratory facilities, and as the laboratory work is expensive and time-consuming, these are available only in relatively few centres.

● Insemination is unlikely to work in the first month. For the sperm to have a chance of being at the right place at the right moment, insemination may be done two or three times each month. Most couples who succeed with AIH do so only after several months of insemination. Many couples find AIH so frustrating and invasive of their sex lives that they may give up after three or four months.

Treatment for the woman

Failure to ovulate

Treatment to restore ovulation is mostly very successful. Unless your ovaries no longer have any eggs in them (premature menopause), modern drug therapy has at least a 90 per cent chance of producing regular ovulation. Unfortunately, for reasons that are not fully understood, probably only 65 per cent of women whose ovulation is successfully induced achieve a pregnancy.

Clomiphene

This is the commonly used fertility pill, normally marketed as Clomid or Serophene. Clomiphene is a very interesting compound. It was originally developed in an attempt to find a better contraceptive pill, one that did not have the side-effects associated with oestrogens. Clomiphene is technically an anti-oestrogen, with some of the properties of those hormones. When it was found that, when it was given to experimental rats, they still got pregnant, it was shelved. Some years later, a laboratory worker noted that the rats that had been given it were perhaps rather more fertile than average, and further tests were done. Eventually, in 1961, Dr Greenblatt and his colleagues working in the United States produced an epoch-making study of the value of clomiphene for woman who fail to ovulate. Since then this drug has been responsible for more pregnancies in infertile patients than probably any other treatment in the world.

Clomiphene is an ideal, first-line treatment. It is cheap and free from major side-effects. It rarely causes multiple births because it is only a weak stimulant. It is thought to promote ovulation by stimulating the natural release of FSH from the pituitary. This makes the ovaries work harder and produce follicles..

In a way, clomiphene is a victim of its own success; it is too frequently given when it is not appropriate. Too many doctors prescribe it without making a diagnosis first. This has two drawbacks. First, it may delay finding the true cause for the infertility. Second, it can actually be contraceptive, which, you will recall, is why it was first developed. Because it is an anti-oestrogen, it can thicken cervical mucus, making the cervix unresponsive to sperm. It also appears to interfere with the uterine lining, which may prevent the early embryo implanting. These two points, plus the fact that occasionally clomiphene can make the ovaries cystic, are important reasons why this drug should only be taken when there is a genuine ovulation problem, and only under proper supervision.

How is clomiphene taken? Usually, you take one tablet (50 mg) every day for five days, starting from the first or second day of your menstrual cycle. If your cycle is much longer than 28 days, you may be given clomiphene from the fifth day for five days. The dose may be increased (two tablets daily, usually taken together) if you do not respond satisfactorily. There is no point in taking clomiphene for more than six days in each cycle, and doubling the dose beyond two tablets a day is seldom effective.

Unfortunately, clomiphene is unsuccessful in treating women over 40 years old. In our practice, a live birth has happened only once.

How do I know if the clomiphene is working? You may have symptoms which suggest ovulation – breast tenderness, mid-cycle discomfort in your abdomen, vaginal discharge near ovulation time, and/or painful and more regular periods. None of these, of course, proves ovulation. Your doctor should check occasionally that ovulation is occurring, and the best way to do this is with ultrasound. This not only accurately confirms ovulation, but will also detect any cysts that might form. The alternative – a blood progesterone test – is commonly used but is far from reliable in this situation. This is because clomiphene can stimulate your ovary to produce more than one follicle simultaneously, none of which actually ovulates. The progesterone produced by all these follicles at once may raise the level of progesterone in your blood to an ovulatory value – even though you have not actually shed an egg.

What are the side-effects of clomiphene? Clomiphene has few side-effects, and fewer risks. It can give you hot flushes, the commonest problem. A few women notice increased abdominal discomfort at the time of ovulation; more likely, you may have more painful periods – a sign that the drug is probably working. A few women get frequent or irregular periods – they generally should stop the drug. Any cysts which may very occasionally develop are not serious, but the drug should be stopped to give the ovary a chance to recover.

Some people wonder if clomiphene – or indeed any other drug designed to stimulate ovulation – could deplete the ovaries of eggs and cause a premature menopause. There is no evidence for this. Neither is there any truth in the idea that clomiphene can cause cancer of the ovary or uterus.

If you are unlucky, you may just feel unwell while taking clomiphene. Don' t worry too much about this as there are other, similar drugs that you can take instead: Tamoxifen (Tamofen) and cyclofenil (Rehibin). They frequently do not cause the unpleasant side-effects, but they are more expensive. They both can occasionally cause cysts, though.

How long should I take clomiphene?   This is very difficult to say. I personally cannot remember many women becoming pregnant if they have not conceived after nine ovulatory months on clomiphene. Of course, if clomiphene does not restore your ovulation, you should stop taking it sooner.

Human chorionic gonadotrophin (HCG) injections
HCG is similar in chemical structure to luteinizing hormone (LH). You will recall that LH rises just before ovulation, triggering the release of the egg. HCG used to be prescribed with clomiphene; it was taken at mid-cycle to mimic the natural LH release so that the follicles, which have been stimulated by clomiphene, release the eggs they contain. There is now evidence that, unless injections are very carefully timed using blood tests and ultrasound, the HCG will have no useful effect. Indeed, given at the wrong time – say, more than 6–10 hours before or after – it might even interfere with the production of a fertilizable egg. This is why fewer doctors now recommend its use with clomiphene. It has very little or no value on its own.

Bromocriptine (Parlodel)
These tablets are useful if the level of the hormone *prolactin* in your blood (*see* p. 125) is raised and you are not ovulating. Parlodel has also been prescribed in the past for unexplained infertility. This is no

longer done – there is no evidence that it is helpful unless you have high prolactin levels. If this really is your problem (and it is not very common), bromocriptine is a highly effective treatment.

It does have side-effects in some people. Apart from feeling rather unwell, they may feel faint or dizzy and occasionally nauseated. You should not drive a car during the first few days after starting bromo-criptine; I have known one patient (in the early days of the use of this drug) who actually passed out 24 hours after starting this drug. Unfortunately, this happened while she was at the wheel of her car; luckily nobody was hurt. Of course, a complete faint is very unusual.

Human menopausal gonadotrophin (HMG)

HMG (most commonly marketed as Pergonal or Humegon) is a mixture of the pituitary hormones LH and FSH, which stimulate the ovaries. Actually, the active ingredient is FSH – the LH content is not specially therapeutic in this context, but it is expensive to produce pure FSH. HMG is highly effective but very powerful and must be given under close supervision. Generally speaking, it is reserved for cases where clomiphene has failed. However, in certain women, it may be a first-line treatment – particularly if they are not having periods.

An important step in the research on human pituitary hormones was the recognition in 1960 that, during the menopause, the pituitary pours out large amounts of these hormones in an attempt by the body to stimulate the flagging ovaries. This excess LH and FSH spills over from the blood into the urine. In his original research Dr Donini in Rome processed 17,600 gallons of menopausal women's urine – Italy, of course, was a good source as there are large numbers of menopausal women living together in nunneries. This has been an excellent way of making HMG, but if you think about it, it is a bit ironic as this drug is now mainly used for IVF treatments – a therapy which is banned by the Roman Catholic Church.

HMG is given by injection from the early part of the menstrual cycle until ovulation is imminent – usually about five to ten days later. When ovulation is just about to occur, a triggering injection of human chorionic gonadotrophin (HCG) is given as, without this, the ovary will not usually shed the egg. This treatment is quite frequently used for women who are not having any periods at all. In this case, it is quite usual to stimulate a period first by giving the woman some progesterone pills.

Why women on HMG need careful monitoring   Treatment with HMG involves very careful control. It is usual to do daily ultrasound measurements of the follicles in the ovaries, and frequent assays of blood oestrogen are carried out by most clinics. There are two reasons why it is dangerous to take HMG without this close monitoring. First, some women overreact and their ovaries become very enlarged and cystic – the so-called *hyperstimulation syndrome*. Apart from being painful, this can be quite a serious condition and may require in-patient treatment in hospital. Second, because HMG frequently results in the ovary producing more than one follicle, each with its own egg, there is a serious risk of multiple ovulation. Indeed, nearly all the modern examples (much vaunted in the press) of serious multiple births – that is, triplets, quadruplets and quintuplets – have occurred after this treatment. Monitoring helps avoid this problem. If too many follicles are seen on ultrasound, the triggering dose of HCG can be withheld.

If you have been infertile for many years, the advent of triplets may seem wonderful. Believe me, it is not. Multiple pregnancy is much more tiring and dangerous for the mother, carries a serious risk of miscarriage, stillbirth and early loss of the babies and presents couples with great difficulties in the first year or two after birth. Any pregnancy involving more than twins is best avoided if at all possible. Fortunately, with proper care, these complications do not occur.

How long is it worth trying treatment with HMG?   HMG is an expensive drug, and the proper monitoring for it complex. We find that it costs approximately £120 for one month's supply of the drug, and because we believe in very careful monitoring, we probably spend at least another £250 in monitoring each cycle. The total cost in a well-run unit, then, is likely to be more than £350 per month. Consequently, most clinics offer treatment for only three months at a time. At the end of that period, the treatment needs careful review. Frankly, if you have not conceived after definite ovulation in each of six cycles with HMG, you have a less than 10 per cent chance with the treatment if it is continued.

Pump therapy   In a normal person, both FSH and LH are released from the pituitary gland in pulses. There is not a steady stream of production, but rather intermittent bursts occur at intervals of every

140

60–90 minutes. Why this is so is not understood. However, it is thought by some that, as these gonadotrophins are naturally produced in this way, it would be more physiological to inject HMG in similar pulses.

To save the poor patient an injection every hour, she wears a little battery-operated electric pump attached to a syringe. This can easily be strapped to an arm, and is soon forgotten. Every 90 minutes or so (the interval can be varied), the little pump does its work and a small amount of hormone painlessly enters the bloodstream. There is an impression that pump therapy may help ovulation, particularly in some cases of polycystic ovary disease.

Pure FSH treatment

During the past few years, pure FSH has been available. Initially, there was great excitement about it as it was widely expected to be much more effective than HMG. In fact, pure FSH (brand name Metrodin) has proved to be a disappointment. It is as good as HMG, but no better, except in certain specific and unusual cases. Because it costs three times more than HMG, it should not be used for the routine induction of ovulation. However, recently we have had some success with a special low-dose regime with this drug; this is not as expensive and may have a place for women with polycystic ovaries.

Treatment with releasing hormone (LHRH)

The normal production of the pituitary hormones LH and FSH depends on the secretion of releasing hormones from the hypothalamus in the brain. Just as LH and FSH are produced in pulses, so is the stimulus from the hypothalamus. In 1979, it was shown that the injection of LH-releasing hormone (usually called LHRH) in regular pulses could produce ovulation. This treatment is particularly useful when the communication between the hypothalamus and pituitary gland is not working normally. It involves the woman wearing a pump (like the pump therapy described above), which injects the required amount of releasing hormone at regular intervals.

LHRH therapy has less risk of producing a multiple pregnancy than does treatment with pituitary hormones. This is because the pituitary is left to work on its own and can regulate its activity depending on how much hormone the ovaries actually need.

141

Drugs which stop the pituitary gland from working

In the last few years, there has been a significant break-through with drugs which "freeze" the pituitary gland. The discovery and synthesis of LHRH led to the development of compounds that are chemically similar and which have powerful medical applications. The one most commonly used to treat infertility is buserelin (Suprefact).

Buserelin currently comes in the form of a nasal spray. Because it is short-acting, it needs to be taken every four hours, and last thing at night and first thing in the morning. There are other, longer-acting drugs being developed which will be less inconvenient, but so far there has not been adequate time to prove their safety. When buserelin is first given, it stimulates the pituitary to produce more FSH and LH. This effect only lasts a day or two, following which the production of these two hormones falls dramatically and stays low. Long-term (more than a few days) administration of buserelin there-fore results in the ovaries becoming inactive – no longer stimulated by the pituitary hormones. Oestrogen production falls to low levels. In effect, a woman taking buserelin becomes menopausal – a very strange treatment, seemingly, for somebody wanting to get pregnant.

However, once buserelin has suppressed the ovaries, they are very receptive to gonadotrophins such as HMG, given by injection. The latest research shows that sometimes the eggs which are produced by this method are of "better quality" and more likely to produce a suc-cessfully growing embryo. Moreover, the ovaries seem able to produce more eggs simultaneously when buserelin is used, and this may be of particular benefit during IVF treatment (*see* p. 165).

Buserelin treatment with HMG is now being used for women who respond poorly to HMG alone and not at all to clomiphene. It probably is most suitable for those who have polycystic ovaries. If this is your problem, it may well be worthwhile asking your consult-ant more about it.

Progesterones

Some women are said to have a "deficient luteal phase" when the ovary does not produce enough progesterone after ovulation. It is claimed (there are many arguments against this) that this leads to the endometrium being underdeveloped and incapable of receiving a fertilized egg satisfactorily. Some doctors give progesterone, usually by injection or by a vaginal pessary, in the hope of a better environment developing inside the uterus. Others give injections of HCG which stimulates the ovaries to produce their own progesterone after ovulation. There is very little evidence that these treatments work.

Surgical wedge resection of the ovaries

Many years ago, before the powerful drugs that stimulate ovulation were developed, it was discovered that removing a piece of the ovary surgically could actually help ovulation, and that this treatment worked particularly well in some forms of polycystic ovary syndrome. It used to be thought that the effect was produced by breaking the thick ovarian capsule, which subsequently allowed the trapped eggs to escape. However, this operation fell into disrepute, partly because it involved opening the abdomen and partly because it tended to cause adhesion formation, which could prevent the tubes from functioning properly.

There has, however, been a recent revival of interest in this operation, for two reasons. First, by using microsurgery or a laparoscope the risk of adhesion formation has been abolished. Second, it has been found to be effective in some women when all drug treatment has repeatedly failed. It now is thought to work possibly by altering the powerful growth factors in the ovary, which can change the growth of the follicles. Seven of our patients have become pregnant after this operation in the last two years.

Dealing with a pituitary tumour

Rarely, a very raised prolactin level may mean a benign tumour of the pituitary. Most of these respond to drug treatment alone, using bromocriptine. Occasionally, however, the tumour may be too large for this and, if left untreated, could affect eyesight. A hospital CAT scan may be requested. This is a special computerized X-ray, which will give information about the size and position of the tumour. If it is very large, your doctor may advise surgery. Rest assured, this kind of pituitary surgery is not life-threatening. It generally results in a woman not producing enough pituitary hormones, but these can be replaced by drugs. I have seen many successful pregnancies following this surgery and treatment with hormones.

Tubal damage and adhesions in the abdomen

Treatments for disease of the Fallopian tubes, or for adhesions in and around the tubes and ovaries, involve some form of surgery. Until about 1970, tubal surgery was well known to have abysmal results. A survey of the world literature showed that, if the tubes were completely blocked, no more than about 10 per cent of women had a live baby following surgery. Even when the tubes were damaged but not blocked, surgery to release adhesions (when internal organs have become stuck together) gave, at best, no more than about a 25 per cent chance of a live baby afterwards. Naturally, this dismal record greatly influenced many infertility specialists. Many gave up surgery completely. Others invariably advised women to avoid having tubal damage corrected. Tubal surgery was left to a handful of enthusiasts, who continued to do their best.

The internal diameter of the human Fallopian tube is very fine. At the tube's narrowest point the fertilized egg goes through a tunnel less than 0.4 millimetres in diameter – the thickness of a piece of thick thread. Hardly surprising, then, that operations to join up this portion of the tube, performed with the naked eye alone, were so unsuccessful. It was only when operating microscopes became widely available and were adapted for abdominal surgery in the 1970s that tubal surgery became a viable option for women with blocked tubes. Within a few years, success rates were doubled, trebled or even quadrupled in some cases. Regrettably, in the United Kingdom, where the treatment was pioneered, microsurgery has been slow to be properly implemented. Consequently, some women still get operations which fall well short of the ideal.

What is tubal microsurgery?

Microsurgery is any form of surgery involving the use of a microscope and very fine instruments. Nearly all patients with pelvic adhesions or damage inside the abdomen causing infertility also have some damage to their tubes – hence the word "tubal". Tubal microsurgery is a term which is loosely used to include not only operations on the Fallopian tubes but also those on the ovaries, or even sometimes the uterus. In my view, virtually all operations in a woman's pelvis should involve the use of a microscope. These tissues are extremely delicate and easily damaged. Adhesion formation, which can make some severely infertile, is very common after operations using conventional methods and not the specialized equipment which is essential for the best results. Unfortunately, once a woman has developed adhesions following naked-eye surgery, adhesions can be extremely difficult or even impossible to treat.

What operations are done and how successful are they?
The following are the most important and frequently performed operations.

Division of adhesions   The most common operation is division of adhesions around the tubes, ovaries or the uterus. The technical term is *adhesiolysis*, or *salpingolysis* if the tubes are involved. These operations do not always need a microscope, but the surgeon should always employ some form of magnification, perhaps with magnifying spectacles. Success rates vary between 30–65 per cent, depending on the degree and extent of adhesions. Operations for adhesions following previous surgery give much poorer results. The success rate when magnification is not used is less than half that obtained following microsurgery.

Opening the ovarian end of the tubes   Approximately 65 per cent of all tubal blockage involves the delicate, finger-like extentions of the outer end of the tube, the *fimbria*, which are near the ovary. The fimbria are responsible for picking up the egg. When this end of the tube is blocked, fluid fills the tube and a swelling called a *hydrosalpinx* forms. The operation to open the tube is known as a *salpingostomy*. The success of this depends on (1) the degree of damage an (2) whether a microscope is used. The results gleaned from the world scientific literature show that when the naked eye is employed for salpingostomy only 8 per cent of patients later conceive; with the microscope, up to 40 per cent of them do.

If the tubes are fibrous (thickened with scar tissue) or the tubal lining is very flattened and damaged (usually diagnosed with a careful X-ray), tubal surgery of any kind will give very poor results and we prefer to offer IVF. About 8 per cent of all pregnancies after salpingostomy (including those resulting from IVF treatment) end as ectopic pregnancies (*see* Chapter 13).

Opening the uterine end of the tubes   This is one of the great success stories of modern infertility treatment. Until the microscope was employed for this operation in 1975, the standard operation was *tubal implantation,* in which the blocked part of the tube was removed and the remainder of the tube was implanted in the uterus through a new hole bored into its wall. With this only four surgeons in the world reported a reasonable number of operations where more than 20 per cent of the patients later conceived, but with micro-surgery, between 45 and 65 per cent of women have a live baby.

The modern operation is called *cornual anastomosis*, in which the blocked part of the tube is removed and the remainder is stitched back on to the original opening. It is difficult technically and fairly time-consuming, but the surgical effort is certainly worth it, particularly as the ectopic pregnancy rate afterwards is only about 3 per cent.

Reversal of sterilization   A few women bitterly regret their decision to be sterilized. If you are unfortunate to be in this position, you probably will recall that your decision was possibly taken at a moment of great stress and pressure, or at least when your circum-stances were substantially different. Microsurgery has been highly successful in reconstituting tubes which have been previously cut or tied. If sterilization has been done with a clip (a frequently used method), reversal is very likely to be possible. Overall, success rates vary from between 65 per cent and 95 per cent, largely depending on the experience of the surgeon, whether a microscope is used, and the type of sterilization being reversed. However, surgery is not a satis-factory option if nearly all of both tubes have been badly damaged or removed.

What does this surgery involve?
Tubal microsurgery tends to take a bit longer than conventional surgery – in skilled hands no more than an extra 30–45 minutes – but you will not feel worse after surgery because of this. On the contrary, because this surgery is done with delicacy, most patients recover far quicker than after conventional procedures. Nearly all surgeons now use a "bikini" incision – that is, a cut in the skin which goes across the pubic-hair line, and which leaves only a very faint scar after six months. Most of my own patients usually remain in hospital for about five days afterwards, but different hospitals may have different routines. There is some discomfort, but never unbearable pain. The most common problem is "wind", with swelling of the abdomen which can be very uncomfortable for about two days afterwards.

What happens after tubal microsurgery?
The first major event, which so many people worry about quite need-lessly, is removal of stitches, usually done on the seventh day after

the operation. This takes only a few seconds and is painless – surprising how many people panic.

The real path to recovery takes place after stitch removal. Obviously, the way individuals tolerate surgery varies. You may find that you are ready to go back to even quite energetic work within two weeks of leaving hospital. Equally, you may take much longer to recover fully. It is very usual to find that you are much more tired than normal for at least four or five weeks after tubal surgery.

At first, it is reasonable not to strain your abdomen. You need not worry too much about this; the importance of not carrying heavy weights is probably greatly exaggerated. It is wise not to strain yourself too much for the first two weeks after leaving hospital, because this can delay wound healing and make your abdomen very sore. Coughing, or straining when you go to the toilet, may make you feel apprehensive – and perhaps quite sore – but causes no problems. Remember, it is virtually impossible to damage the surgery on the tubes themselves, no matter how much you strain.

Sex after surgery Basically, this can occur as soon as you both feel like it. You cannot harm the operation, nor will you block your tubes. It may simply be the last thing on your mind when you leave hospital, though you may feel very different 10–14 days later.

The unofficial world record for post-surgical sex is, as far as I know, held by a 27-year-old American. I operated on Jane on a Wednesday, opening both tubes in a $2\frac{1}{2}$-hour operation, through quite a large hole in her abdomen. Late the following sultry Saturday afternoon, 75 hours after waking from anaesthesia, the ward nurse, a rather shy girl, was doing her rounds. Entering Jane's side-ward, she saw our patient and her large Texan partner in an extremely interesting position. Nursing manuals do not give much advice about what to do in situations like this. Jane had a positive pregnancy test 16 days later. A letter she sent me recently tells me that her little boy is exceptionally good at sport.

Seeing your doctor after microsurgery Regular clinic attendance is, I think, essential after tubal surgery. We like to see all our patients every three months until they get pregnant, or until they decide to give up or to try alternative treatments. This allows us to do a good deal of fine tuning – such as rechecking ovulation, the sperm counts and generally ensuring that fertility is maximized.

Should you have any gynaecological symptoms after surgery, I strongly advise that you see your doctor promptly. It is possible to get further inflammation or infection, and this needs the promptest treatment. If you think you may be pregnant, by even a few days, you should seek medical advice. There is a somewhat higher risk of ectopic pregnancy once your tubes have been cleared after surgery(*see* Chapter 13), and your doctor may suggest an ultrasound examination and routine blood tests to exclude this.

If, after about a year of trying, you still have not become pregnant, a laparoscopic examination is very worthwhile. This will confirm whether or not the tubes are still in good condition, and whether or not you have any adhesions. Some clinics do an X-ray – but this does not give nearly as much information, and risks your developing more inflammation. If you are older than average – say, more than 36 – it may be worth having a laparoscopy earlier than one year after surgery, so that you can decide whether or not to enter an *in vitro* fertilization programme.

Your feelings after a tubal operation   Women vary in how they feel after tubal surgery. Some feel much more optimistic and, if they don't get pregnant, come to terms with it. Others, especially if they have not been carefully advised beforehand, expect to get pregnant immediately and feel increasingly let down and anxious when they have a period each month. Be warned: Tubal surgery does not often work immediately, and unless you remember this, you may end each month feeling quite devastated when your period starts, particularly if it happens a day or two late. Following any fertility surgery, there is a 10 per cent chance of conception each month at best. It is essential, therefore, to get things in perspective.

Emma is a well-to-do housewife. Both her tubes had become blocked near the uterus following an infection after a miscarriage. I performed cornual anastomosis surgery when she was 34. She was very depressed when she did not conceive immediately, even though I felt the operation had gone really well. Within three months of surgery, she became increasingly concerned and tearful and asked to be treated by *in vitro* fertilization. At that time, IVF was even more unsuccessful than it is now, and I refused her as gently as I could. She immediately referred herself to another unit, and over the next two years, had four unsuccessful treatments with IVF, never really giving herself a chance to come to terms with her problem. She then returned to our clinic and had extensive counselling and joined our support group. Three years after the operation, she had her first baby, James; since then she has had another boy and, ten months ago, a baby girl.

What about the laser to unblock my tubes?

There has been a huge amount of publicity about the use of lasers in surgery generally, and for infertile patients particularly. Many advantages are claimed for tubal microsurgery using lasers, including less blood loss, more accuracy in cutting, greater speed and less adhesion formation. In fact, the only advantage that is not claimed for laser microsurgery is that there is a better chance of pregnancy if the laser is used.

My own bias is that the laser is not particularly useful for any tubal surgery when the abdomen is opened. I actually find the surgery takes me longer with a laser, and that healing is no better than after fine microsurgery with diathermy (when blood vessels are sealed with the heat from a high-frequency electric current); consequently, we stopped using the laser some time ago. Certainly lasers are very useful for the treatment of pre-cancer of the cervix. However, there is no evidence that the chances of pregnancy occurring are higher with laser, and this lack of evidence, rather than the expense involved, has persuaded the National Health Service in the UK that extra lasers are not needed. Perhaps the only real justification for the use of lasers in tubal surgery is during laparoscopy (*see below*).

Surgery done down the laparoscope

In recent years, there has been considerable interest in surgery done during a laparoscopy. The laparoscope is introduced in the usual way, through a small hole in the navel. One or two small cuts about $\frac{1}{4}$ inch (6.4 mm) in length are made in the abdomen low down near the pubic-hair line and fine instruments are introduced through these holes. Long fine scissors or tweezers can be introduced and adhesions cut. Some surgeons even feel confident enough to open the ends of the tubes, if they are blocked near ovaries. Cutting has to be done with some care, and all blood is continuously washed off the tissues using a fine jet of fluid also introduced through the abdominal wall. This can then be sucked out with a small tube. Bleeding can be controlled using a special diathermy machine.

Some surgeons, particularly in the United States and France, use a laser beam as their main instrument during laparoscopic surgery. They claim that this gives better control over bleeding, which is probably true. Whether the cutting is more accurate I rather doubt. The percentage of women becoming pregnant afterwards is quite

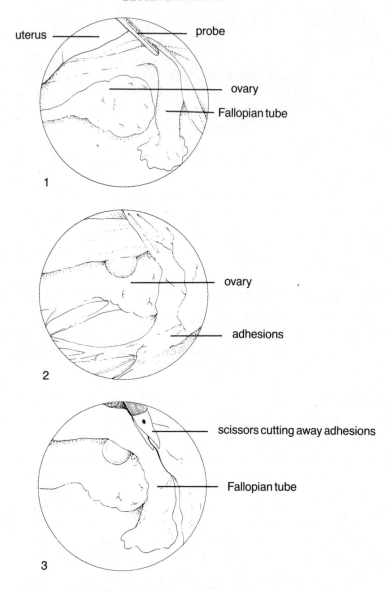

Division of adhesions using the laparoscope. The laparoscope is first inserted through the navel; afterwards, small scissors on a probe and sometimes forceps as well, are inserted through the skin above the pubis. (1) Surgeon's view of a normal right tube, ovary and part of the uterus — no division is required. (2) In another patient adhesions surround the right tube and ovary. (3) These adhesions have now been treated by the scissors and the picture much more closely resembles the normal view.

good, but there are no proper studies comparing laser laparoscopy with conventional laparoscopic surgery, nor has anyone yet shown that laser laparoscopy gives better results than open microsurgery.

The main advantage with laparoscopic surgery, whether done with a laser or not, is the rapidity with which women recover. Usually only a single overnight stay in hospital is required, and there is no abdominal wound which takes time to heal. Results are best in experienced surgical hands.

The success rates with this kind of surgery are claimed to be high, probably as good as open microsurgery. Unfortunately, laparoscopic surgery is not always possible.

Some doctors suggest "hydrotubation" – what is this?

Following tubal surgery of any kind, some doctors recommend passing fluid under pressure into the tubes to keep them open. This is called *hydrotubation* and is done by passing saline (salt water), or a similar fluid, through the cervix and into the tubes. A few doctors even try to unblock the tubes by this method, rather than employing surgery.

There is no evidence that passing fluid through the tubes is a useful treatment. Nor is passing gas, which is still a treatment used in a few clinics. Nor does it give any useful diagnostic information, unless done at the time of X-ray or laparoscopy. Hydrotubation can be painful, and there is a risk that you might get a tubal infection. It has little or no place in modern therapy.

Passing balloons or dilators into the tube

Some doctors have recently begun to use fine dilators (or balloons), which are passed through the uterus into the tube, to treat blockage where the tube joins the womb. It requires the use of X-rays to guide the surgeon, and can be done without an anaesthetic. It is similar to the recent invention of angioplasty – when radiologists pass thin tubes into blood vessels in the heart to widen them and prevent angina and heart attacks. It may have an application in fertility surgery – certainly it saves hospital admission – but there is, as yet, little evidence of its value since there have been few pregnancies.

Treating endometriosis

Treatment for endometriosis (*see* p. 88) is a very controversial issue. Some doctors feel that endometriosis never causes infertility, except when it causes severe distortion and scarring of the tissues, or when it results in bad adhesions around the tubes and ovaries. Others believe that even mild endometriosis should be treated, because it may cause infertility, and it may get worse and cause bad scarring and distortion, with tubal and ovarian damage. I personally am firmly in the "no treatment" camp, except when there is clearly severe distortion, or if a woman is suffering pain or discomfort – a common symptom. If you are to have treatment, what is available?

Laparoscopic surgery with or without the laser

Spots of endometriosis can be burned with diathermy or laser, during a laparoscopy. The advantages are that it can be done at the time a diagnosis is made, it does not require major surgery and, unlike drug treatment, it does not stop you ovulating. However, there are a number of disadvantages: it is expensive, and not always available; it must be performed while you are under a general anaesthetic; and there is absolutely no evidence to show that you are more likely to conceive afterwards.

Drug treatment

Drug treatments depend for their effect on the fact that endometriosis, like the endometrium (womb lining), is hormone dependent – that is, it grows when there is enough oestrogen around. Therefore, the aim of all drug treatment is to reduce the amount of oestrogen in the body and thus cause the endometriosis to stop spreading and perhaps shrink.

The most widely used drugs are probably the contraceptive pill and progesterone-like drugs. They damp down your ovarian activity and the endometriosis melts away. Another commonly used drug is danazol (Danol), which is a compound that resembles testosterone (male hormone) and which also markedly reduces ovarian activity. A third group of drugs, recently introduced, are the LHRH analogues (buserelin is one example; *see* p. 142). These produce a temporary menopause, and the endometriosis shrinks away.

The advantages of drug treatment for endometriosis are that no surgery is needed, any pain is always improved and it may prevent the spread of endometriosis. However, some women feel very unwell on these drugs, you can't get pregnant while taking them and the endometriosis tends to regrow as soon as you stop treatment.

Microsurgery

One reasonably effective way of dealing with endometriosis is to remove it surgically, and it is probably the best way of stopping its recurrence. Unfortunately, when endometriosis is very extensive, it is often not feasible to remove all the affected tissue, nor all the active areas of endometriosis; neither is the use of a microscope particularly helpful. Conversely, open surgery is not justified if the disease is mild.

With microsurgery, you can try to get pregnant immediately you recover. In addition, it is the only reliable way of treating endometriosis that is causing cysts on the ovary, and it is the best chance to prevent a recurrence of the disease. On the other hand, it does involve an operation and your being out of action for about three weeks. It can also make adhesions worse, especially if the procedure is done in an unskilled fashion, and you may find that the pain caused by the endometriosis may not have improved.

All treatments for endometriosis carry about a 65 per cent chance of pregnancy at best. If the endometriosis is extensive, the success rate will be considerably less. Occasionally I get the strong feeling that women become pregnant in spite of the treatment – certainly if mild endometriosis is left untreated, your chances of pregnancy are as good as if it is treated.

In vitro *fertilization or GIFT*

This may occasionally be justified when endometriosis is causing infertility (*see* Chapter 11). It tends to be less successful if the ovaries have endometriotic cysts, and these may need surgical treatment first.

Problems in the uterus

Uterine problems may require a surgical approach. Many of these operations are relatively minor, and can be done on an out-patient basis. A few are occasionally treatable with drugs.

Fibroids

Fibroids (*see* p. 76) can certainly cause infertility if they are close to the uterine cavity and distort it, or if they displace the ovaries, or if they grow close to where the Fallopian tube enters the uterus, causing a blockage. Treatment is generally surgical. The operation to remove fibroids is called *myomectomy* and is fairly similar to tubal microsurgery.

The fibroids are removed from the uterus, usually after cutting into the uterine muscle. If you can imagine cutting cleanly into a peach to remove the stone, without disturbing the flesh of the peach too much, you will get some idea of what is done. Following removal of the fibroid, the space where it lay is carefully stitched together, and the muscle of the uterus is also repaired with stitches.

The uterus has a fairly good blood supply and may bleed during the procedure. This is why it is usual to make sure that some blood of your blood group is on hand in case the bleeding is vigorous. This is just for safety's sake – in practice, a blood transfusion is very rarely needed.

When this operation is done in women under the age of 35, about 65 per cent will conceive. It is much less successful after this age, with only about 35 per cent becoming pregnant.

Congenital abnormalities

Perhaps the most important of these is a *septate uterus* (*see* p. 90). This can usually be dealt with by simply cutting it using an hystero-scope (telescope inside the uterus). This is a very effective treatment and can usually be done with no more than an overnight stay in hospital. There may be a little vaginal bleeding afterwards, but usually no more than during a period. If the septum is very large, your doctor may prefer to remove it by opening the uterus from above and performing an operation rather like removal of a fibroid. The chance of a pregnancy afterwards is about 75 per cent.

An uncommon abnormality is a *double uterus*. This may be repaired by joining the two halves of the uterus together. This kind of surgery is rather specialized and is best done in a centre where a good deal of this work goes on. Unfortunately, if the operation goes badly, it can' t easily be changed later. Properly done uterine reconstruction of this sort (called *utriculoplasty*) carries a 65 per cent chance of pregnancy.

The third abnormality is a *rudimentary or non-functioning uterine horn*. This is usually the second, less well-formed half of a double uterus. It may justify removal, in which case open surgery will be needed.

Internal adhesions (synechiae)

These cause the walls of the uterus to stick together and can usually be separated by a fairly simple vaginal operation. Sometimes the surgeon may use a hysteroscope and a special pair of scissors. Recently, some doctors have experimented very successfully with the laser. Although the operation can be done as a day-case, usually under quick general anaesthesia, it frequently needs to be repeated. One or two of our patients have needed five of these little operations spaced over several months. Fortunately, there is no pain.

Sometimes it is necessary to place a plastic coil (an IUD) in the uterus for a few weeks after this operation to help to keep the uterine walls apart. Antibiotics may also be given, and sometimes steroid and oestrogen tablets, all of which help the healing process. The chance of a pregnancy after this operation is about 70 per cent.

Polyps

Nowadays, this is really about the only serious indication for an infertile woman to have a D & C (dilatation of the cervix and curettage), or "scrape". Removal of a large polyp – which is not very common – gives a good chance of pregnancy on the rare occasions when it is the cause of the infertility.

Adenomyosis

This puzzling condition, where the uterus becomes increasingly scarred following invasion of its muscle wall with lining tissue, is very difficult to treat. As we have seen with endometriosis (*see above*) the endometrium (or lining tissue) is sensitive to the ovarian hormone oestrogen. If the level of this in your body is reduced, the lining tissue is reduced as well. The usual treatment, therefore, is the same as drug treatment for endometriosis. This damps down your hormones and will control painful or irregular periods, but it will not help you get pregnant. Surgery will not help either. Generally it is impossible to remove the adenomyosis without damage to the uterus. Fortunately, this condition is uncommon, and only a few women become infertile as a result of it. If you have adenomyosis, you probably have about a 35 per cent chance of getting pregnant.

Problems with the cervical mucus

Just how important cervical mucus problems are is difficult to say. Certainly, there is probably as much nonsense written about cervical mucus as there is about any other topic in infertility. However, there seems little doubt that if the post-coital test is persistently negative, the outlook for a baby is less. We have tried various treatments to improve the acceptability of sperm to the cervical mucus, but we have been disappointed. Sometimes we find that the test becomes positive and, within a few cycles, there is a pregnancy. However, there is little good evidence that these women would not have got pregnant without the treatment.

Douching with bicarbonate of soda

Many women are advised to douche with a weak alkali, such as bi-carbonate of soda, to soften the mucus and to correct the acidity of the vagina. The belief is that the sperm are being killed off by acid vaginal secretions.

This advice is fallacious as all women normally have an acid vagina. This is nature's protection against infection. Moreover, the sperm stay in the cervical canal inside the mucus, which is not acid and which is generally not affected by the vaginal fluid. There is no evidence that any form of douche improves a woman's fertility.

Oestrogen tablets and vaginal creams

Oestrogens help the cervix to produce great quantities of watery mucus. This does seem to improve the post-coital test in some people, and pregnancies are reported, but we do not know whether the apparent improvements in cervical mucus are the real cause of these pregnancies. Taking oestrogen in small doses (even by a cream in the vagina) can help some women ovulate, and it could just be that the pregnancies which seem to occur with oestrogen therapy happen because of improved ovulation rather than improved mucus.

Steroid tablets

Cortisone-like drugs may be given if you have antibodies attacking the sperm as they enter the mucus. Although there is some evidence that this may be of benefit, my own feeling is that it is not really safe for a woman to take steroids for this purpose. A short course of two or three weeks at a time might be reasonable, but long-term steroid treatment can cause stomach ulcers, changes in the bones with loss of calcium, emotional disturbances and increased susceptibility to infection. Steroids are probably best reserved for life-threatening diseases.

Cryotherapy or laser treatment

One theory is that abnormal (sperm-resistant) mucus is made by abnormal cervical gland cells, and if these are frozen, or burned, normal surface gland cells will tend to grow in their place, and this will promote the production of good mucus. There may be some truth in this, but no really good trials of either laser treatment or cryotherapy (when the cells are frozen) have ever been conducted. At least these treatments are painless and cause little or no serious inconvenience. They can be done during a simple visit to your clinic.

Antibiotic treatment

It has been said that one reason why the cervix may not let the sperm survive is because of infection. Various bugs have been incriminated. It has been fashionable to blame chlamydia, mycoplasmas and ureaplasmas, partly because these ill-understood bacteria are often found on the cervix. Unfortunately for the pundits, these bacteria may also linger in the cervix and vagina of normally fertile women. Some years ago, a very clever study was done which showed that whether you had treatment for these bacteria or not made absolutely no difference to your fertility. In fact, women who were not treated actually got pregnant faster. This has not stopped many doctors from continuing to give women drugs against these infections.

More importantly, many women who are infertile worry greatly that a thrush infection or an infection with trichomonas, both of which are very common in the vagina, is preventing them from getting pregnant. This worry is quite without foundation, unless of course, symptoms from the infection (such as soreness) are preventing them from having intercourse.

Artificial insemination with your partner's sperm

Generally speaking, there is usually little point in artificial insemination with your partner's sperm (AIH). This bypasses the cervix by putting sperm directly into the uterus, but there is very little evidence that it will do much good. My feeling is that your partner can do that perfectly well himself and usually with much greater pleasure for both of you.

There is a very important point here. Repeated post-coital tests and inseminations may well be more than you feel like bearing. Most people find it very unpleasant to have sex "to order", and regular attendances to have insemination by a white-coated doctor can greatly interfere with your self-esteem and your sex life. All of us repeatedly see women conceive without any treatment, in spite of many negative post-coital tests.

157

CHAPTER TEN

Unexplained Infertility

Unexplained infertility is a matter of considerable argument. It seems extremely unsatisfactory to label a couple as suffering from "unexplained infertility". Some textbooks and articles even give it a name – "idiopathic infertility" – as if this makes it respectable. Of course, all that "idiopathic" means is "unexplained". In reality, our labelling infertility as unexplained simply means a failure by the experts to find the cause.

Some clinics calculate that as many as 25–30 per cent of their patients suffer from unexplained infertility. My own view is that, if the doctor looks hard enough, a clear cause for the infertility can usually be found. This may mean doing very careful tests, and sometimes even repeating tests. At Hammersmith, we calculate that only 5 per cent of our patients truly have unexplained infertility.

Why does all this matter? There are basically three reasons:
- First, when the cause for the infertility is not available, treatment cannot be rational. Various "remedies" will be tried on a purely haphazard basis. Consequently, luck will play a greater part in whether or not the woman gets pregnant.
- Second, there will be inevitable pressure to turn to the "high tech" treatments, particularly IVF or GIFT, in the hope of striking lucky. This involves the couple in complex and demanding medicine, which may delay a correct diagnosis and more effective treatment being commenced.
- Third, infertility is emotionally taxing. It is very much easier to come to terms with your infertility, even if you never conceive, if you can find out what has been and is causing it. A "diagnosis" of unexplained infertility throws an extra psychological burden on a couple.

What are the likely causes of "unexplained" infertility?

We have recently completed a survey of our patients with unexplained infertility, who had been infertile for a minimum of three years. Some had been trying for a baby as long as 17 years; all of them had seen at least one specialist and had been advised to try a "high tech" treatment such as IVF.

Each of these couples was carefully reinvestigated. The preliminary results make interesting reading because, in about 80 per cent of cases, we felt we could identify a clearly treatable cause for the infertility. At the time of writing this study is still in progress. What we can say is that many of these couples with an identified cause for their infertility have since undergone quite simple, but specific, treatments of various kinds and already more than one-third of the women are pregnant or have delivered, without recourse to IVF. The following are the most common problems we found.

● *An unexpected problem in the man.* Although all the men had initially had normal sperm counts, when the sperm were subjected to a separation test (see p. 119), we discovered that many semen specimens showed subtle but important abnormalities. Moreover, we confirmed that, when the separation test improved, a pregnancy often occurred soon afterwards – frequently within two or three months. Conclusion: About 30 per cent of unexplained infertility is due to poor sperm function.

● *A problem in the uterus.* Many women with unexplained infertility had not had the uterus properly evaluated. Many had not had an X-ray (hysterosalpingogram; in other cases, the X-ray was not of good enough quality to make a proper diagnosis. On careful re-evaluation, we found a high proportion of women had fibroids, polyps or adhesions in the cavity of the womb and adenomyosis. Approximately half of those treated for fibroids, polyps or adhesions conceived; adenomyosis treatment gave very poor results. Conclusion: About 20 per cent of unexplained infertility is due to a significant uterine problem.

● *Subtle problems with ovulation.* Many women turned out not to be ovulating every month, or to have subtle problems associated with their hormones. We found that several of the women we examined using the ultrasound machine had polycystic ovaries, but it is uncertain whether or not this was causing the infertility. Some of these women had a poor response to drugs to stimulate ovulation when being treated by IVF. Conclusion: At least 15 per cent of unexplained infertility is associated with abnormal hormone secretion, which affects ovulation.

• *Tubal problems and endometriosis.* A surprising number of women had some degree of tubal damage, which showed up on a repeat laparoscopy or hysterosalpingogram. In some cases, there was clear evidence of scar tissue in the portion of the tube where it joins the uterus. Other women had quite marked endometriosis which presumably had developed (or got much worse) since a previous laparoscopy. Open surgery produced several successful pregnancies, even in several cases when IVF had already failed. Conclusion: About 15 per cent of unexplained infertility is due to tubal damage, or to severe endometriosis which has been difficult to identify at an earlier laparoscopy.

• *Cervical problems.* Many couples had never undergone a post-coital test; alternatively, a negative post-coital test had been ignored or not followed up. Some of these women undoubtedly had a problem with their cervical mucus. Repeated tests were negative; in some cases, treatment resulted in the test becoming positive, although pregnancy rates remained rather discouragingly low. Conclusion: Some unexplained infertility may be due to a problem with the cervical mucus, though the precise importance of this is unclear.

• *A genetic problem.* Several couples had an abnormal chromosome analysis. This affected either the man or woman and could not be treated directly. Furthermore, unexplained infertility may also result from a gene defect when the chromosomes *look* normal but carry an abnormal gene that cannot be detected. Conclusion: At least 2 per cent of unexplained infertility is due to a genetic defect.

What tests should be done if the infertility is unexplained?

I would strongly recommend that every reasonable effort be made to establish a diagnosis before complex treatments, such as IVF, are undertaken. Here is a list of the tests most commonly forgotten. Some may well be worth carrying out for the first time or repeating if there is still doubt about the diagnosis.

For the woman

● *Good X-rays of the uterus* – hysterosalpingogram (HSG) – are really worth getting. The HSG gives information about the womb and, to a lesser extent, the tubes which cannot be obtained by laparoscopy alone.

● *Hysteroscopy.* If there is any suspicion at all of an abnormal uterus, a telescope inspection of its interior is well worthwhile. Sometimes this reveals abnormalities that do not show well even on X-ray.

● *Carefully timed post-coital tests are often forgotten.* They help to establish (1) whether there may be a sperm problem, (2) whether there are antibodies to sperm in the cervical mucus and (3) whether there may be other problems in the cervix itself preventing manufacture of good mucus.

● *Repeated laparoscopy.* If a year or two has elapsed since the last inspection by laparoscopy, it may well be worth repeating it. If it is, it should be done by somebody with a keen interest in infertility. Photographs should be taken so that there is a permanent record of what exactly was seen.

● *Thorough hormone tests* done throughout the menstrual cycle. A study we have just completed shows that routine, single plasma progesterone tests – the most common test for ovulation – are only reliable 65 per cent of the time. Regular blood samples – perhaps taken every day around the mid-cycle – may be needed to see if there are any subtle problems which might either affect ovulation or the quality of the eggs produced.

● *Ultrasound scans* of the ovaries. These should be done at the beginning of the menstrual cycle – requiring possibly four or five tests – to confirm that ovulation is really occurring and that there is no sign of polycystic ovaries.

For the man

● *Repeated sperm counts,* over several months if necessary. Far too many men have just one count done. This is not sufficient for any serious investigation of infertility and certainly not enough if there is a somewhat obscure cause for it.

● *Sperm function tests.* Several different tests are coming into regular use. They include the sperm separation test (see p. 119) and the hamster test (see p. 121), but I am not convinced of the latter's reliability. Alternatively, some hospitals are now doing special examinations of sperm under an electron microscope. This powerful machine magnifies much more than a conventional microscope and may help to find a problem in some of the sperm.

For both partners

● *Chromosome tests* on both partners to see if there is any abnormality which might prevent a normal embryo being formed.

All these tests are well worth considering if you have been told that your infertility cannot be explained. Certainly you should discuss them with your doctor, and if they can be done, I suggest that you make every possible attempt to establish the cause of the infertility as clearly as possible. In the next chapter, I discuss IVF and GIFT, treatments which are frequently offered to people with unexplained infertility. Both are stressful, emotionally demanding and physically invasive. Moreover, they are usually quite expensive. Before undertaking either of them you should first try to establish the cause of your problem.

Thirty-nine-year-old Kathleen had been told by several doctors that her infertility was unexplained, and she was advised to have IVF and/or GIFT treatment. Because she was desperate (her marriage was not secure) and because she was quite well off, she underwent no fewer than seven attempts at IVF and three at GIFT in the next two years. All this treatment was done privately, and she tells me that in two years, she spent a total of £25,000. In all that time she never had an X-ray of her uterus to see if the cavity was normal. When I suggested this, the subsequent X-ray showed a large polyp. She came into hospital for the day and it was removed in an 8-minute procedure. She conceived two months later.

CHAPTER ELEVEN

Test-tube Babies and Similar Treatments

What is the test-tube baby technique?

Test-tube baby treatment is the process by which egg and sperm are mixed outside the body and then returned to the womb after fertilization. It involves the removal of an egg from the woman's ovary, the collection and purification of sperm from her partner, the mixing of sperm and egg in the laboratory and, if fertilization occurs, the insertion of the developing egg – the embryo – into the woman's womb. The embryo is placed in its mother's body usually two days after fertilization, while it still consists of only a few cells and long before any organs have started to be formed.

What are "*in vitro* fertilization", "extra-corporeal fertilization" and "embryo transfer"?

"*In vitro* fertilization" (IVF) really means fertilization in glassware (from *vitrum*, Latin for "glass"). "Extra-corporeal fertilization" is another term, mostly used by those too obstinate to employ the more widely accepted terminology; it merely means fertilization outside the body. "Embryo transfer" is the process of placing the embryo into the mother's uterus.

Many people confuse "artificial insemination" with the test-tube baby technique, but it is totally different. In artificial insemination, a doctor or nurse places sperm directly into a woman's vagina, cervix or uterus using a syringe or other artificial method, rather than conception occurring by natural intercourse. However, fertilization occurs within the woman's Fallopian tube in the usual way.

IVF is supposed to be very successful. If it is, why bother with other infertility treatments?

One of the most unsatisfactory aspects of IVF, and, indeed all the newer reproductive techniques, is the way in which they have been promoted. In the 12 or so years since Louise Brown, the world's first test-tube baby, was conceived most ordinary people, many journalists and not a few doctors have come to believe that IVF has been the greatest step forward in infertility treatment. This impression is really utterly wrong; as we shall see, the reality is quite different. IVF is still the most demanding, the most emotionally fraught, the most expensive, and the least successful of all infertility treatments. More importantly, it is also one of the least available or accessible.

What is the evidence? Whichever way its success is examined, one has to say that IVF results are still very disappointing. In Britain each year, the Voluntary Licensing Authority for Human *In Vitro* Fertilization and Embryology (VLA) officially collects and collates the results from all the IVF clinics in the country. There is no doubt that its report is accurate. The latest (at the time of writing), published in May 1989, gave the following statistics for the preceding year:

- only 10.1 per cent of all treatments produced a live baby.
- IVF units treating fewer than 300 women annually were even less successful than this.
- fewer than 7,500 women in the whole of Britain were treated by IVF.
- five IVF centres in Britain were responsible for the majority of the pregnancies and the remainder were, by and large, less successful;
- only 650 babies were born following IVF or GIFT.

What do these statistics mean? There are thought to be more than 5 million couples of child-bearing age who are not using contraception in Britain. Statistics also suggest that one in ten of all couples are infertile. Potentially then, there are at the very least 500,000 infertile couples in Britain, yet only 7,500 of them even received IVF treatment last year (one in 100) and only 760 babies were born to them following IVF (1 in 750, counting twins as a single birth). In addition, although nowadays it is extremely difficult to adopt a baby in Britain, almost twice as many couples successfully adopted than had a baby born by IVF. Perhaps this, more than any other statistic, focuses attention on just how unsuccessful IVF really is.

In view of all this, you may appreciate why I believe that the wide press coverage given to IVF is so unfortunate. As I have stated, it is one of the least successful of all infertility treatments, and promotion of it has taken attention away from other treatments which are usually far more helpful. A fraction of the investment given over to IVF would, if spent in other areas of infertility, undoubtedly produce more babies. Many academic units of obstetrics and gynaecology argue that they pursue IVF because of its value in research. Actually, remarkably little valuable research emanates from the majority of IVF units, academic or private.

In my opinion, test-tube baby treatment is, with a few notable exceptions, the last resort, useful only when a diagnosis indicating it has been firmly established or when all else has failed. Even then, it is quite definitely *not* suitable for *all* cases when other treatments have failed. At Hammersmith Hospital we only offer this treatment if there is some chance of success, however small. We feel very strongly that other treatments, being generally more successful, must usually be tried first, and that IVF should be reserved for when there is no realistic alternative and after every attempt has been made to establish a cause for the infertility.

The stages of IVF treatment

(1) Testing your suitability before treatment

From what I have said, it must be clear that IVF is by no means suitable for every infertile couple. This vital aspect is often ignored. About half the women referred to IVF programmes would be much more appropriately treated by a different technique. Therefore, before treatment is started, several sperm counts, tests to discover your hormone levels and other procedures should be carried out to confirm whether you have a chance of success. For example, the condition of the uterine cavity should be reviewed (perhaps by X-ray) if this has not been done recently; it is most important to make sure that the womb is healthy enough to allow an embryo to implant and develop. The woman might even be given drugs to make her ovulate so that her response to these drugs can be assessed well before an actual treatment cycle. This enables the medical team to tailor treatment to suit your individual needs.

(2) Stimulation of ovulation

The best chance of successful pregnancy is obtained when more than one embryo is placed in the uterus at the same time. This is because so many early human embryos, normally fertilized, are lost or do not develop into babies. Consequently, one way of overcoming this natural tendency is to put back several embryos simultaneously during IVF. When two, three or even four embryos are put back together, the risk of a multiple pregnancy such as twins is not as great as you might expect, though it is certainly high enough to be a cause of real concern.

In order to obtain more than one embryo simultaneously, more than one egg is needed. This is why drugs such as clomiphene (Clomid) or HMG (Pergonal) are given to make the ovaries work harder than normal. Occasionally, many eggs are obtained simultaneously with these drugs but it is very uncommon for all of them to fertilize and form into embryos.

One of these drugs will normally be given to the woman (in the form of either an injection or pills) a few days after her period, at the start of the treatment cycle. The dose and the length of time these drugs are given may be deliberately varied, depending on her individual response. Recently, many IVF centres have been using so-called "programmed cycles". This ensures that the doctors have a greater degree of control over the ovaries, just temporarily, which may allow more precise timing of when eggs should be collected. The evidence suggests that this approach can improve the results of IVF. Many clinics are also giving the drug buserelin (Suprefact) in addition to HMG. As we have seen (p. 138), buserelin prevents the pituitary gland from sending messages to the ovaries, and this means that the ovaries respond more effectively to the HMG treatment given subsequently. This seems to result in more eggs being produced simultaneously, with a higher pregnancy rate in certain cases. Other clinics use progestogens (synthetic forms of progesterone), which are cheaper and may give comparably good results.

(3) Assessing the development of the eggs

Egg collection is generally timed to within a few hours of when the woman is expected to ovulate. If eggs are not collected very close to this time, they may not fertilize properly. This is the main reason why so many tests are often done to confirm the status of the woman's hormones and, thus, development of her eggs.

There are basically three ways by which the chance of collecting mature eggs can be improved. None is wholly accurate, and a good deal of experience and some informed guesswork is used to pinpoint the moment before ovulation.

• *Hormone tests.* As the follicle swells, the hormones oestrogen and progesterone are produced in increasing amounts. Regular blood tests can detect this increase. Also, provided the woman is not taking the buserelin, the pituitary gland in the brain produces luteinizing hormone (LH), which gives a message to the ovary to start the ovulation process. This hormone can also be detected in the blood.

• *Ultrasound.* The swelling follicle can be directly measured using ultrasound (*see* p. 123). This is usually done daily. We know from experience that, when the follicle is about 20 millimetres across, ovulation is imminent. Ultrasound performed through the abdominal wall requires a very full bladder, and this can be remarkably uncomfortable. Recently, more clinics have started to use vaginal ultrasound – the ultrasound probe, instead of being placed on the abdomen, is inserted gently into the vagina. We find that most of our patients greatly prefer this: they can take an intelligent interest in what their doctor is seeing on the screen, without bursting to go to the toilet.

• *Injection of HCG* shortly before ovulation would normally occur. This gives a message to the ovary to initiate the chemical processes in the egg which occur when a woman ovulates. It is usually only used if the pituitary gland has not yet started to produce LH or if the woman is taking buserelin.

(4) Egg collection.
Eggs may be collected by laparoscopy, in which case a general anaesthetic is given. More usually, the eggs will be collected using ultrasound, and often with vaginal ultrasound. In this method, a needle is placed through the top of the vagina and into the ovary, and eggs sucked out from the follicles. This is a very convenient technique, frequently involving only a light anaesthetic or merely a little local anaesthetic with sedation. We find that most of our patients much prefer this approach. If local anaesthesia is used, the woman has to be in hospital for only a few hours.

In spite of the great care that is taken, it is not always possible to get all the eggs (or sometimes even a single egg). However, in good centres, 97 per cent of attempts at egg collection yield at least one egg – so the risk of total failure at this stage is small.

(5) Egg culture, sperm preparation and fertilization
Once the eggs have been collected, they can be easily damaged. They are carefully identified under a microscope in the operating theatre

suite and then immediately placed in specially prepared fluid. This fluid – the culture medium – contains very precisely measured amounts of the chemicals needed for the eggs' survival as well as some of the woman's own serum previously obtained from a routine sample of her blood.

The eggs in their culture medium are then put into an incubator. This is simply a kind of oven, which will keep the eggs at exactly the right temperature under rigidly controlled conditions which resemble those within the body as closely as possible.

Usually shortly before the eggs are collected, the man will be asked to produce semen by masturbation. A bedroom is available in most clinics for this purpose. Men often find this aspect of IVF very worrying – it is quite common to find that a man simply cannot ejaculate under this kind of emotional pressure. If this is likely to be a problem, most good units will make arrangements to carefully freeze and store samples of the man's semen, ready for use well before the treatment week. Unfortunately, semen that has been frozen and then thawed is not usually as fertile as freshly produced semen.

Once the semen has been produced, the sperm are washed and diluted in the laboratory, and the number of sperm are counted under a microscope. Several hours after egg collection, they will be mixed with the culture medium containing the eggs and these will then be replaced in the incubator. Unfortunately, it is not uncommon to find a last-minute problem with the sperm: they may be too few in number or too weak in other ways. At present, most IVF programmes need several thousand normal sperm to guarantee fertilization of even a single egg.

(6) Embryo culture

In a good IVF unit, the cultured eggs will be inspected under a microscope about 18 hours after they have been mixed with the sperm, and again after about 24–30 hours. The reason for the inspection at 18 hours is that this may be the only time that definite signs of fertilization may be observed. The egg may actually divide into several cells later on, without ever having been fertilized. This is called *parthenogenetic cleavage* (*see* p. 32), and in clinics that are not very efficient, there is risk that unfertilized, parthenogenetically cleaved eggs may be transferred to the womb. These, of course, give no chance of normal pregnancy.

The embryo will usually have divided into about 2–4 cells after 48 hours, although occasionally growth may be more advanced than this. Before an embryo is transferred to the womb, the scientists check to make sure it appears normal. If there is doubt about this, they may suggest waiting for a further 24 hours before a decision is taken about its transfer. If an embryo seems seriously abnormal, it is discarded, rather than run the slightest risk of a defective infant.

(7) Embryo transfer

When an embryo is ready to be put back into the womb, it is loaded into fine plastic tubing, together with a minute drop of culture fluid. After the woman is vaginally examined briefly, the tubing is inserted through her cervix. The fluid containing the embryo (or embryos, if there are more than one) is now squirted extremely gently into the womb. This is normally very easy indeed and, as it is painless, hardly ever requires an anaesthetic. Most clinics usually put the embryos into the womb with the woman lying on her back, but on rare occasions, she may be asked to kneel. Which way is required largely depends on the position of the cervix and uterus. Once the embryo transfer has been done, most clinics ask the woman to remain lying down for a few hours, or even possibly overnight. It is thought that this may help the embryo to "stay put", but there is no good evidence for this.

Injections (or suppositories) of progesterone are frequently given to the woman after embryos are transferred into her uterus. This is thought by some to help a pregnancy to implant, but there is much doubt whether it really helps you to get pregnant. IVF programmes which have stopped this treatment do not seem to do any worse than those that continue it.

At this stage, once an embryo has been transferred, nearly all women are naturally nervous about what they can or cannot do. Immediately after embryo transfer, many are so anxious that they might damage the early embryos that they lie rigid in bed for hours at a time. This is quite unnecessary – all that is wanted is for you to lie down for a couple of hours to help you relax. Remember that, in any case, embryos do not immediately implant after transfer – this takes place several days later, and there is no evidence that this is influenced by routine activities. If implantation was influenced by a woman moving around, then clearly none would ever get pregnant, particularly if energetic sexual activity took place. You should not regard yourself as an invalid, but perhaps it is not unreasonable to

169

take it easy for a few days. We suggest that our patients stay off work for two or three days and avoid having sex for two weeks. There is categorically no need to stay in bed. However, there is no evidence that even these simple precautions make much difference. On the other hand, overseas travel is best avoided for two weeks, if possible, if only because you may want to keep in close contact with the clinic that treated you.

(8) Pregnancy testing

Although everything up to this stage may have gone quite easily and embryos were put into the uterus without difficulty, the chances are high that the woman will not get pregnant. Many embryos are lost before the menstrual period is due, and this can be extremely disappointing. The reasons for these failures are not clear.

Some clinics do not test for pregnancy at all; others suggest that the woman sends them a urine sample if she wishes. We normally take some blood from all patients on the 7th, 12th and the 14th day after embryo transfer – the earliest that a very small pregnancy can be detected.

IVF and male infertility

There are a number of techniques that have been attempted to overcome a low sperm count. Several units have tried placing the eggs in very small volumes of fluid with the sperm. This technique may help fertilization rates by concentrating all the available sperm closely around the egg. Other units have had very limited success with fertilizing eggs in tiny droplets of fluid containing sperm which has been taken by needle aspiration from the man's epididymis. At present, such a sophisticated approach is very experimental.

Sperm injection into the egg

There has been great interest recently in attempts to improve fertilization rates by manipulating egg and sperm together during IVF treatments. Two main approaches have been employed by research workers around the world. The first has been to dissolve the outer shell of the human egg – the *zona* – using enzymes or acid solutions. This has the theoretical advantage that sperm which are not very motile, with help, might be capable of penetrating the softer, "business" parts of the egg and forming an embryo. Embryos have resulted from this method, but there is a question mark over their normality. Total removal of the zona may leave the egg so unprotected that it could become infected with viruses; this would be highly undesirable as it perhaps just could lead to an abnormal baby. Another problem is that we do not know whether a reasonably intact zona is required for normal embryonic development.

Because total removal of the zona seems essentially unsafe, other workers have tried drilling microscopic holes in the zona. It is thought that sperm might get through these holes rather more easily than through zonas that are intact. Researchers have been successful in getting such eggs to fertilize. However, fertilization has been pretty erratic, and to date no human embryos have formed successful pregnancies as far as I am aware.

An alternative approach has been the deliberate injection of sperm into the egg, using a sophisticated microscope and micromanipulators. The egg is quite invisible, so such microsurgery requires quite complex equipment. The egg is immobilized by suction from an extremely fine pipette, and a minute stab wound is made with a remarkably fine glass tube. A single sperm is chosen and then injected into the egg. Animal pregnancies are reported with this technique, and several human embryos have been formed leading, in one or two cases, to successful human pregnancies. However, there is still a long way to go before this could become a clinically useful treatment. One of the problems is that we have no idea how to select a healthy sperm for injection; this technique may force an unhealthy sperm into an egg with unforeseen results.

When should IVF be considered?

The main situations where IVF may be worth considering would seem to be:

● When the tubes are badly damaged and tubal surgery has less chance of success than IVF, or in most cases where tubal surgery has already been unsuccessful. In both these situations, IVF should be considered because it bypasses the Fallopian tubes.

● When the man's sperm count is on the low side or abnormal, yet potentially capable of fertilizing sperm. Here IVF may be useful because fertilization can possibly be manipulated and observed by the scientific team.

● For certain women who have problems with the cervix, perhaps "hostile" mucus. IVF bypasses the cervix and its mucus.

● For women who are not ovulating spontaneously, but who

produce eggs on fertility drugs without conceiving. In this situation, the ability to force the ovary to produce many eggs and then select the best ones for fertilization and transfer means than IVF may be a suitable option.

● For some women with endometriosis or those with very carefully investigated infertility which remains unexplained. Here the supposition is that either fertilization or proper implantation of embryos is not taking place.

● Most recently, for certain couples who are at high risk of having genetically abnormal babies.

Who is unsuitable for *in vitro* fertilization?

Unfortunately, there are many women with damaged tubes, or who have one of the problems listed above, for whom even IVF is of no help. These include woman who:

● have had the womb removed (*hysterectomy*).

● have severe scarring or abnormalities of the womb (such as bad adenomyosis), making pregnancy impossible.

● have had tuberculosis (or another serious infection) of the womb which has left scar tissue.

● have very scarred or extensively cystic ovaries. It may be impossible to collect a healthy egg, even though there may be circumstantial evidence that ovulation is occurring.

● have very severe bowel adhesions around the ovaries which could make even ultrasonic egg collection very dangerous.

● are much over 41 years old – when IVF is notoriously unsuccessful.

In addition, IVF is generally unsuitable if the man's sperm count is lower than 100,000.

What are the chances of success?

At the present time, at the best clinics in the world, up to 45 per cent of women having an embryo transfer get pregnant, and no more than 15 per cent miscarry. Unfortunately, most units do not do nearly as well as this. In general, if you have had only one embryo transferred, your chance of a pregnancy will be about 12 per cent; with two embryos, it will be closer to 24 per cent. The more embryos transferred, the better the chance of a pregnancy. The problem with transferring many embryos is the risk of multiple birth.

What factors are associated with IVF success?

What causes success in some cases and failure in others is not known. However, certain factors are associated with a normal pregnancy after IVF. These include:

- Transfer of more than one embryo simultaneously.
- The age of the woman. Those over 38 do less well. If a woman does get pregnant at 40 by IVF, the chance of a miscarriage is much higher than normal.
- Careful hormonal measurements. Careful control of hormone levels gives a better chance. Many test-tube baby programmes do rather limited hormone testing. The advantages of doing fewer hormone tests are that this makes the treatment cheaper and that the woman has far fewer tests interfering with her life. The disadvantage is that the success rate may be lower. Moreover, if the eggs fail to fertilize and tests have not been done, it may not be possible to say whether they failed to fertilize because the hormones were just not adequate in that cycle of treatment, or whether there was some other problem – for example, with the sperm. This can be a big problem if further treatment is subsequently considered.
- The ability to collect eggs around the clock, seven days a week. Although this puts a huge strain on the staff and requires special efforts, the ability to collect eggs night or day, holidays included, has advantages for the woman.

What are the reasons for failure?

Even when patients are selected carefully, there are many pitfalls. Failure can occur at any stage. Unfortunately, the further that treatment has proceeded, the harder it is to accept failure, particularly if everything had seemed to be going well. The reasons for failure include:

- The ovaries may not produce a suitable follicle or follicles in the cycle during treatment. Alternatively, one of the ovaries may become enlarged temporarily with a cyst. If either of these things happen, treatment may have to be abandoned. In most cases, it will be possible to restart treatment after a period of resting the ovaries. Between 8 and 20 per cent of treatment cycles are abandoned, depending on the programme, so this is quite common.
- Eggs cannot be collected from the follicles at the time of laparoscopy or ultrasound. This accounts for less than 5 per cent of failures.
- The eggs fail to fertilize. This occurs in about 20–25 per cent of

patients. Your partner's sperm may just not be healthy enough on the day of egg collection; this can happen even when many previous sperm counts haven't revealed a problem. Unfortunately, male infertility is almost certainly the most common reason for IVF to fail totally.

● The embryo or embryos fail to develop normally and have to be discarded. Perhaps 20 per cent of embryos fall into this category.

● An embryo or embryos are transferred to the uterus, but they don't implant. This is the most common reason for failure, occurring 70 per cent of the time. Just why apparently entirely healthy-looking embryos don't implant is still something of a mystery.

● The embryo implants and pregnancy commences, but a miscarriage occurs within a few weeks. Alternatively, in 6 per cent of cases, the pregnancy lodges in the tube (an ectopic pregnancy) from where it needs to be removed surgically. The incidence of miscarriage varies greatly from clinic to clinic – usually somewhere between 15 and 30 per cent.

What are the risks of *in vitro* fertilization?
Will my baby be normal?
At the time of writing, over 8,000 babies have been born following IVF, and they show that there is no special risk of abnormality. Approximately 1 in every 50 babies born as a result of natural intercourse have an abnormality of some sort. This risk is not increased after IVF; indeed, there is some evidence that certain types of abnormality (such as chromosome problems – Down's syndrome, for example) are actually less common after IVF. There have been suggestions that test-tube babies tend to have more problems at birth and that stillbirths are very slightly more common. In fact, this apparent trend is not due to the IVF but probably because many infertile women (who end up with successful treatment) are in the "high-risk" group.

Is there a risk of twins or triplets
It is difficult for IVF to be successful unless more than one embryo is transferred simultaneously, but the more embryos that are transferred at once, the greater the chance of twins, triplets or even more. This is why the number of transferred embryos should be limited. Many infertile women, after years of forlorn treatment, are only too ready to accept such risks, but although a twin pregnancy is

not too difficult to deal with, triplets are undoubtedly best avoided, and quadruplets or more are really a disaster. Apart from the risks of a premature delivery, bringing up so many babies at the same time places a great burden on a family. The best IVF units will always limit the number of embryos transferred simultaneously, even if this means a slightly reduced success rate. Actually, good units (perhaps because of their control procedures and the quality of the embryos they produce) seem to need to transfer fewer embryos to get good success rates.

Is there any physical risk to the woman?

Very occasionally the drugs given to stimulate the ovaries may cause too many follicles to develop. This may result in the ovaries becoming temporarily swollen and cystic – the so-called hyperstimulation syndrome – a condition which often requires hospital admission but usually settles down after a few days' bedrest. The main risk is associated with egg collection, which, however trivial, is still a surgical procedure. Most people are pretty scared of anaesthesia, but because virtually all IVF units are in very sophisticated hospitals or clinics, you can be reassured about this. If you have ultrasonic egg collection, this is no more risky than a laparoscopy.

Will we be able to stand the emotional strain?

In vitro fertilization is very demanding emotionally. Both women and men always find it more stressful than they expect. Having to go to the hospital regularly, the inevitable waiting around, travelling and staying away from home, the monitoring of follicle growth all result in tension and worry. The build-up to laparoscopy or ultrasonic egg collection, with the possible admission to hospital and the waiting time until embryo transfer (assuming this is possible) require considerable fortitude. In addition, it is often not easy for the man to produce his semen at the moment of egg collection. Once the embryo has been put back in the womb the situation can be even more fraught because the chances are about even that the woman's period will come on within the next two weeks. Not infrequently, this occurs after a delay of a few days or so and, of course, this can be quite devastating.

These real problems are a fact of treatment, and it is most important that couples should only enter treatment if they feel strong enough to bear these kinds of shocks and the waiting that it involves. It is also important that couples should support one another; many find an added strength in their relationship at times like this.

Can the treatment be repeated?

This largely depends on your response to your previous treatment attempt. It occasionally becomes clear that no amount of hormone therapy or treatment for deficiencies in the sperm (both relatively common examples) will make IVF successful. Under these or similar circumstances, IVF should probably not be repeated. Sometimes such decisions can be re-evaluated months or even years later, if there have been any hopeful scientific or medical developments. Most clinics will repeat the treatment for suitable patients, although some set a limit of about three or four attempts. In the private sector, it generally depends on how you feel and if you and your partner are confident that you can stand the upheaval – and if you have the money!

How much does it all cost?

Most IVF in Britain is performed on a private basis; only a very few units are wholly or partly funded by the National Health Service. IVF may be available in a few teaching hospitals on a semi-private basis. However, the money charged by these units often goes to help patients who cannot afford private fees and to pay for research. Without research, IVF will never improve, and because of this these units are often very deserving of your private fees and support. It seems regrettable that, far too often, couples are prepared to pay for IVF at private clinics until their money runs out, and then come to these very hard-pressed academic units demanding treatment.

How to choose an IVF clinic

Once you have decided to go for IVF, you may have great difficulty in choosing a good IVF clinic. There are several ways in which people may get information, none of which is always completely satisfactory. They include:

● *Referral by your family doctor or a gynaecologist at a local hospital*. Some people rely on what their GPs or their gynaecologists tells them. Sadly, many family doctors and, incidentally, very many consultant gynaecologists do not check out thoroughly the IVF clinics they recommend to patients. They usually have very little personal experience of IVF and may actually be in a far worse position than you to make a proper rational decision. While I still think that a doctor's referral is best, our profession undoubtedly needs to try harder to get really accurate information about suitable IVF clinics, so that patients have the best choice.

● *The media.* Some people are heavily influenced by what they read in the press, but they are quite often wrong to do so. For example, *The Independent*, normally an excellent newspaper, has published a list of British IVF clinics with the services each offers; moreover, this guide includes data on success rates, which normally you might think was the best yardstick of all. Unfortunately, claimed success rates are not always verifiable. A clinic that is not very successful, and which relies on its income from private practice, is hardly likely to publish success rates which are less good than those of its competitors. This has been pointed out in the medical press in an honest and impressive letter by one of Britain's most respected IVF scientists, Dr Simon Fishel from Nottingham. His contentions are borne out by the fact that some success rates claimed in the aforementioned survey look rather better on paper than in practice. This is why at least one leading responsible clinic has refused to advertise in this newspaper's survey. I believe that press reports are generally the worst way to get accurate information about any IVF clinic.

● *Self-help or counselling organizations.* The two best organizations in Britain are CHILD and the National Association for the Childless (*see* p. 245), both of which run excellent nationwide networks which provide advice and information including a list of IVF clinics. Inevitably, the information in this list is based entirely on what they have been told by the clinics, but at least they have sufficient experience to be wary of the exaggerated claims which can surround some work in this field.

None of these three alternatives is ideal by any means. If I were in need of IVF, there would be certain points about which I would like reassurance before committing myself to a particular clinic. For what they are worth, here are some of them:

● Did you like and feel confident with the team of doctors and nurses you met there? Did they seem like a team? Do they get on with each other?

● Before treatment, does the clinic carry out adequate tests to establish the diagnosis as precisely as possible? This may seem impossible for you, a lay person, to decide, but it is fairly simple to find out whether they bother to take a womb X-ray (hysterosalpingo-gram, or HSG) when needed, or examine personally X-rays taken earlier at another hospital. Do they also do other ancillary tests, such as a post-coital test, before committing you to IVF?

• Do they have an independent counsellor available for your special problems? By "independent" I mean not someone on the medical staff who is involved i.. the actual treatments. An independent coun-sellor can stand outside your treatment and help you focus on what may be best for you and your partner.

• Do they offer only IVF, or are all infertility treatments properly done? Clinics which focus on IVF as their sole or main treatment tend to offer this to the exclusion of other treatments. This is convenient for them, but may not be in your best interests.

• Who do you know who got pregnant there? This may seem a re-markably silly question – but in the United States, there are over 260 IVF clinics and over half of them have yet to produce a baby!

• Who do you know who failed treatment there and yet were satisfied with what they were told and how treatment generally went?

• How much monitoring of the treatment cycle is done routinely? Generally speaking, clinics which do regular hormone tests tend to get somewhat better results; they also have a better idea of what has gone wrong if the treatment fails.

• Is there just one fixed drug regime for getting the woman to produce many eggs, or do they tailor the treatment to suit her body and circumstances? On the whole, programmes with fixed regimes get less good results.

• Can they do egg collections (or other treatments) at weekends?

• Do you have a choice of local or general anaesthesia?

• Do they do egg collection by both laparoscopy and ultrasound?

• Do their scientists examine all the eggs 18 hours after mixing them with the sperm? This step is essential to ensure that a dividing egg has actually fertilized (*see* p. 168).

• How many embryos do they routinely put back into the uterus? In general, less good clinics need to transfer more embryos to produce pregnancy rates which approach the results of the better clinics. This is important because the more embryos that are transferred, the greater the risk to the woman.

• How much do they charge? If they are charging much more than other clinics – say, over £1,700 (including the cost of drugs) – they may be overcharging you. If they are charging much less – say, much under £1,000 – they are probably not offering the most effective treatment. To some extent, you get what you pay for – cut-price IVF may offer you cut-price treatment.

• If your treatment fails, will you be able to see the director of the clinic? In good clinics, the director should be available (by appointment) to see couples who have failed their treatment cycle. He should be able to go through your treatment cycle with you, working out what, if anything, went wrong, where improvements might be made and whether a further IVF attempt or other treatment is justified.

• Do they do very careful, repeated assessments of sperm quality before the IVF attempt? A good unit will have a set of precisely worked-out values for sperm quality, and will cancel your attempt if they feel that there is really no chance of fertilization. This is really very important because it is far too easy to try IVF when the attempt is doomed to failure.

GIFT

GIFT – gamete intrafallopian transfer – is a newer treatment than IVF. It involves taking eggs from the ovaries and sperm from the man, mixing them together and immediately placing them in the Fallopian tube of the woman, before fertilization. It is different from IVF because it does not involve the formation of an embryo outside the body – instead, the egg is allowed to become fertilized in its natural environment.

The invention of GIFT treatment should be credited to Dr Tesarik and his colleagues in Czechoslovakia, whose idea it first was. This team transferred egg and sperm into the Fallopian tube of a woman undergoing tubal surgery in 1983. About a year later, Dr Ricardo Asch, working in San Antonio, Texas, reported a pregnancy following this manoeuvre. GIFT has since become very popular, particularly in the United States, because it does not require sophisticated laboratory equipment for embryo culture.

GIFT is different from IVF, though there are similarities. An embryo is not formed in culture, but in the woman's own tubal fluid. This may be an advantage as it is now recognized that the precise needs of a developing human embryo are not fully understood. Consequently, we are unable to mimic the ideal environment for fertilized eggs in the laboratory. GIFT overcomes this problem because eggs and sperm are put straight back into the woman's Fallopian tube. This means, of course, that the tube is not bypassed during GIFT treatment – another difference from IVF – and as a result, GIFT is not a useful treatment when there is tubal disease – the main indication for IVF. GIFT also works best when more than one egg is deliberately collected and placed with the sperm, so, like IVF, the woman needs drug treatment to stimulate the ovaries to produce several eggs simultaneously. The eggs are usually collected by laparoscopy, rather than by ultrasound, because the laparoscope is needed to guide the surgeon when the eggs and sperm are being placed in the Fallopian tube.

When is GIFT indicated?

The main reason for GIFT treatment is when absolutely no cause for the infertility has been found. It may also be used when there is a definite problem with the cervical mucus and post-coital tests are always negative. High success rates are claimed for GIFT by many clinics, but at the best centres, there is no evidence that the results are any better than those for IVF.

The problems of GIFT

GIFT and male infertility

This treatment is being very widely used for male infertility. The rationale is that, by placing the sperm and egg very close together, there may be more chance of fertilization. A major disadvantage of GIFT is that, unlike IVF, we are not able to check to see whether the sperm have fertilized the eggs and have functioned normally.

I have to confess to having quite serious misgivings about GIFT in most instances. We do not know why it works, or even how well it works. It is not clear whether it is the preparation of the sperm, or the mixing of the sperm directly with the egg, or the timed stimulation of ovulation which really produces the increase in pregnancies which is claimed. The particular reasons why I have some concerns are:

● Most couples having GIFT treatment are, except for their undiagnosed inability to conceive, healthy and normal. They undergo a very complex and expensive treatment when there is nothing demonstrably wrong. I cannot help wondering whether a much simpler treatment would be as effective.

● To date, there have been no properly conducted trials of GIFT treatment, comparing it with other simpler treatments or, indeed, with IVF.

● Many women are coerced into this treatment by their own desperation. They often feel that they get inadequate testing and treatment, and expect that this treatment will answer their problem. Many women who have failed GIFT treatment have subsequently conceived with much simpler and cheaper remedies.

● GIFT treatment involves the return of eggs and sperm into the body *before* fertilization. This means that less diagnostic information is obtained than with IVF. With the latter, the couple learn that they can produce an embryo.

● GIFT involves laparoscopy to replace the eggs in the tube. IVF can now be done with ultrasound alone, avoiding the need for a general anaesthetic.

● In Britain, GIFT is being increasingly used in district general hospitals which do not have adequate facilities for arriving at a proper diagnosis or providing comprehensive treatment. It is also being "pushed" very hard by a drug company which has a vested interest in selling expensive fertility drugs. This use of GIFT is detrimental to fertility treatments as a whole because it diverts attention from more important, cheaper treatments.

POST, DIPI, ZIFT and SHIFT

Some infertility clinics are not happy unless they have coined their own acronym. These terms have two things in common – each has been coined by someone eager to be at the forefront of the medical practice of IVF, and none of the procedures they represent has any really proven value. In case you still want to know, these terms are:

POST: Peritoneal Oocyte and Sperm Transfer. In this treatment, eggs and sperm are injected directly into the abdominal cavity, in the hope that the Fallopian tube will pick up any resulting embryo.

DIPI: Direct Intra-Peritoneal Sperm Injection. Sperm are injected through the vaginal wall, directly into the abdomen.

ZIFT: Zygote Intra-Fallopian Transfer. The embryo is transferred directly to the Fallopian tube, bypassing the uterus.

SHIFT: Synchronized Hysteroscopic Intra-Fallopian Transfer. Sperm are transferred into the Fallopian tube via a hysteroscope inserted in the uterus.

CHAPTER TWELVE

Donor Insemination and Egg Donation

W e have seen how inadequate the treatment of male infertility really is. Medical intervention makes a difference in relatively few cases. If treatment fails and the man is proved sterile, there are basically only three alternatives. First, a couple may come to terms with the problem, grieve the loss of childbearing and accept that they will never have children. Second, they may look into the possibility of adoption; unfortunately, this is extremely difficult in nearly all developed countries because there are very few "unwanted" babies. The third alternative is donor insemination with sperm taken from another, fertile, man. I emphasize that donor insemination is an *alternative*. and *not* a treatment for infertility. A couple have to come to terms with their infertility problem before taking this decision.

Just as some infertile men produce no sperm at all (for which, of course, there is no treatment) some women have total ovarian failure – that is, their ovaries are quite incapable of producing eggs. While there is also no treatment for this uncommon condition, an alternative is for them to accept eggs donated from another, fertile woman.

While donor insemination is technically relatively simple, treatment involving donated eggs is more complicated, requiring *in vitro* fertilization. Although these treatments are essentially very different, they both raise similar medical, ethical and emotional issues.

Donor insemination

Until recently, donor insemination was always referred to as "Artificial Insemination by Donor" – or AID. It has now had its name changed so that it will not be confused with AIDS or "Acquired Immune Deficiency Syndrome".

Donor insemination involves taking semen, produced by masturbation, from a fertile donor, who usually remains anonymous. This semen is then inseminated into the vagina and cervix of the woman, at a time in the menstrual cycle when she is judged to be fertile. Commonly, insemination is timed using ultrasound tests or blood tests, but a few clinics are now getting their clients to use the urinary LH dipstick (*see* p. 43). Unfortunately, many clinics use only unreliable temperature charting.

Good clinics usually inseminate on at least two occasions during any one cycle, to give a better chance of covering the fertile period. The insemination, is done as described on pages 133–5.

The main indication for using donor semen is male infertility. Most responsible doctors will not use donor sperm unless there is no chance of a pregnancy by any other method. Donor semen may also be suggested if the man is a carrier of a specific genetic disease: using sperm from a donor free from that particular genetic abnormality allows a couple to have children unaffected by that disease.

Sperm donors

These are generally university students. I get the impression that, in the United States, medical students are regarded as ideal donors, which says a lot about the value judgements of the American medical profession. In Professor Snowden's book *The Artificial Family* he describes the case of Addison Hard of Jefferson Medical College in Philadelphia. Dr Hard wrote to *Medical World* in 1909, claiming to have been involved in the first case of donor insemination in 1884. (We now know he was wrong, p. 189.) A local merchant who was sterile had married a woman ten years younger. The case was discussed in the medical school with the students, of whom one was Addison Hard. The students agreed that semen should be obtained from "the best-looking member of the class" and then inseminated. Hard maintains that this was done while the wife was anaesthetized and that neither the merchant nor his spouse knew about it. After the woman conceived, the merchant was informed but pleaded that his pregnant wife should not be told. The surgeon in charge went to his grave with the secret, but when the merchant's son was 25 years old he was visited by the excessively handsome Dr Hard, who could not resist publishing his experiences.

Donors are screened as carefully as possible for serious illness and infection, and they are normally free from any genetic disease. Attempts are usually made to match the donor's physical characteristics with those of the woman's partner. Height, build, colour of hair, complexion and eyes are recorded and matched as closely as possible, as are ethnic group and religion if requested. Most centres doing this work ensure that the blood group of the donor is also matched to the couple, so that there will be no risk of the baby developing Rhesus disease.

In recent years, there have been huge worries over the problems that AIDS creates. Donors are now screened to confirm that they are free of the virus. Moreover, their semen is held for a period of quarantine: all donor semen is frozen and stored in liquid nitrogen for a minimum of three months so that absence of the AIDS virus can be confirmed. This practice works to some extent against the infertile couple as semen that is frozen and then thawed is not quite as fertile as freshly ejaculated semen. However, it is an essential safeguard. (Some also worry that freezing the sperm may produce an abnormal child, but this is definitely not true.) Opinions vary about whether donors should be paid for their services. Payment certainly introduces a commercial element, with the inevitable risk that an unhealthy donor may be persuaded to sell his semen, perhaps passing on a serious infection. Donors who give away their semen are certainly very altruistic, but this kind of altruism is increasingly rare in our society – particularly if you consider what tests and inconvenience a donor has to experience. A rather poor compromise is usually reached, whereby the donor is paid his "expenses" only.

A second important feature of donors is that they are rarely of proven fertility. Most have never had children nor, indeed, are they in long-term relationships. (If they were, they probably would be much less likely to give their semen because they would begin to understand the implications of giving their genetic material to a third party in this way.) If repeated inseminations with one particular donor's semen fails to produce a pregnancy, most clinics switch to a different donor. Unfortunately, most donor programmes have only a limited number of good fertile donors (especially since the appearance of AIDS) and this inevitably means that semen from one donor is often used for a large number of pregnancies. This has obvious, serious disadvantages. Above all, it increases the risk of two people (both children conceived via donor insemination and therefore both related) meeting in future and having children of their own. This, above all, worries very many religious people. It also has important genetic implications as in-breeding greatly increases the risk of genetic abnormalities developing in the population.

A third feature of donors is that they are virtually always anonymous. This is partly to protect the donor, and partly for the benefit of the recipient. A donor does not want any responsibility for the offspring. There is growing concern about this because recently, in Britain, it has become widely felt that the children who are born following donor insemination should be able to know who their genetic fathers are. The law at present is very unsatisfactory. Most donors would not be prepared to donate if they were required to identify themselves; it has therefore been suggested that the insemination clinics keep non-identifying information about the donors, so that children can at least have some rough idea of what sorts of people their real fathers are. This may also be very important if, for example, the child develops a genetic disease later in life which might be thought to be inherited from the father.

What is very clear is that donors are not properly counselled or even advised about the implications of what they are doing. Donors are usually young, with no ties, and may not fully recognize how they may feel in future about having donated sperm. It is said that many donors, years after donation and perhaps following marriage, worry deeply about their uncertainty as to whether they have children whom they do not know and for whom they can take no responsibility.

In Britain until recently a child born following donor insemination was illegitimate and the so-called "father" had no legal rights. This anomaly in British law has now been rectified by Parliament in the Family Law Reform Act of 1988. The birth certificate may now be signed by the "father" and the child is legitimately his.

Ethnic and religious issues

One difficulty that most clinics have is finding a donor with a specific racial or ethnic background. For example, Asian donors are very difficult to find: few Indians in Britain, for example, will consider

185

donating sperm; and similar difficulties are experienced in getting Chinese donors. This can be very difficult for a couple who are eager to accept donor insemination, but want very much to preserve their own racial and cultural identity.

Insemination with the semen of a known donor

Some couples much prefer to be inseminated with the sperm of a person whom they know. Usually this is a close relative, but occasionally it may be a particular friend. Most medical practitioners are very wary of this as it creates the potential of a new type of family relationship. For one thing, there is always the risk of the donor watching his child grow up under parental guidance of which he disapproves. He may feel very possessive towards the child and attempt to interfere in later life with his or her care or psychological well-being. Such arrangements may also tend to create an unhealthy bond between the donor and the mother. Such a bond could destroy a marital relationship. The other problem is that a child perceives that he or she has, in effect, three parents. This could be very disruptive for the child's proper development, and could cause great distress if he or she felt unhappy with various parental decisions. It is likely that the brunt of these problems would be worst at puberty, when a child desperately needs the background of a stable nuclear family.

Should you consider donor insemination?

The decision to have donor insemination is a very personal one, and nobody can tell you whether or not it is right for your relationship. It is like adoption in many ways, with the advantage that the child will be genetically related to at least one of you. Moreover, donor insemination is much easier to achieve. It is said that, every year, there are well over 10,000 babies born following donor insemination in both the United Kingdom and the United States.

There is something of a stigma associated with donor insemination. Many men are remarkably reluctant to admit that they are sterile, and so they and their partners keep the insemination a closely guarded secret. Friends and even parents – the prospective grandparents – are not told. Certainly, whether you are going to reveal the true origins of your child is something you need to think over very carefully. It is wise, indeed probably essential, to go for professional counselling. There are a number of hospitals and clinics which provide this, and it is also available in the private sector.

Questions that may be asked

Will my partner love a child from a sperm donor?

Women sometimes ask this question, but in my experience, this is not a problem. The male partner becomes deeply involved and shares pregnancy and birth. I have seen so many husbands in this situation made obviously and rapturously happy that I cannot believe that there is a serious risk of estrangement. If the decision is taken mutually and it is freely discussed, the man's relationship with the child should be just the same as that of other children with their genetic fathers. The environment in which we bring up children is, in many ways, much more important for their development than a blood relationship. You can be assured that your child will rapidly take on the characteristics and outlook of your partner and so he will be just as involved in parenthood as you yourself.

Most experts who have studied this aspect of donor insemination find no evidence of any particular problems – either emotional or psychological – within marriages where donor sperm has been used. Dr Margaret Jackson, a remarkably brave and intelligent woman who was perhaps the great British pioneer of donor insemination, felt that, in her experience (which was greater than that of anyone else that I know), marriages where donor semen was used were frequently enriched and improved.

Dr Robert Snowden, a professor of sociology in Exeter and leading expert in this field, who is properly very cautious about donor insemination, agrees that there is evidence to suggest continued bonding between the children and their "fathers". Even when a donor insemination marriage fails, there is good evidence that the husbands often feel the same way about the children and wish to care for them, as if they were genetically their own.

It is worth remembering that there are many fathers who are genetically related to their children, who treat them appallingly. A genetic relationship is no guarantee of family harmony.

Will my child love his/her father?

Everything that I know about donor insemination leads me to conclude that children regard "adoptive" fathers as theirs. Many children in this situation seem to regard their parents particularly highly, because they went through so much to have them. One boy, having had things explained, wrote: "He's my Daddy – I'm just pleased that they loved me enough to be able to share their secret with me and with my sister. I feel tremendous warm love for them both...."

How do you get donor insemination?

Your doctor may well be reluctant to raise the subject at all and you may need to be the one who asks whether this could be considered. Your doctor may then suggest where you might go for this treatment. Donor insemination in Britain is mostly available only privately. There are only 11 clinics in Britain that I know of which offer donor insemination on a National Health Service basis; this is not many when you consider that there are 200 health districts in England and Wales and these few clinics may well be geographically out of reach. Private treatments are not cheap, and are certainly expensive if proper ovulation monitoring is carried out as well. Some clinics screen the recipients very inadequately, even though their donors are properly monitored.

The National Association of the Childless (*see* p. 145) can put you in touch with reliable donor clinics. Another possibility is the British Pregnancy Advisory Service; this is a non-profit-making organization with some 40 branches around the country, some of which provide donor insemination. I do not advise you to go there specifically for in-fertility treatment, however, because it seems to me that this is not always as nearly as expertly carried out as their donor insemination. Similarly, the Family Planning Association may be able to offer you advice as to what is available in your area. It is worth remembering, incidentally, that most clinics, even the private ones, have waiting lists for insemination.

If you do go for donor insemination, remember that this is not nearly as successful as natural intercourse. Usually no more than 50 per cent of women will be pregnant after nine treatments; this means considerable upheaval and expense. It is also worth keeping in mind that donor insemination is not very pleasant emotionally; some women find it very clinical, and, unfortunately, the burden of the treatment is something they cannot easily share with their partners, who are left out by the very nature of what is being done.

One word of advice; if you do go to a private clinic for donor in-semination, do not have endless repeated treatments without getting yourself checked. If you have not become pregnant within four or five months of trying insemination, you should make certain that any fertility tests you have not had done are completed.

An unusual case of donor insemination

Artificial insemination is not so very new. One of the earliest pregnancies achieved by this means was reported in the *Lancet* over 100 years ago, on 2 January 1875.

Dr Capers, an army surgeon, fought with General Grant in the American Civil War. In May 1863 a comrade-in-arms, next to whom he stood in the line of battle, suddenly fell to the earth with a wound from a minnie bullet. Almost simultaneously, Dr Capers heard a piercing scream from a house 150 yards behind. Examining the young man, he found a fracture of the lower leg, but the bullet had "ricochetted from these lower parts and, in its onward flight, had passed through the scrotum, carrying off the left testicle". Dr Capers dressed the wounds, and a few minutes later "the esteemable matron of the house" ran up in the greatest distress to say that her 17-year-old daughter had been badly wounded a few minutes earlier. He ran to the house to find that she, too, had a bullet wound in her lower abdomen. He attended her but thought she would die. The army was forced to retreat; fortunately, the girl recovered and the doctor rejoined his regiment.

Six months later, the fortunes of war found Dr Capers back in the same place. He naturally visited his young patient, who "was in excellent health and spirits, but her abdomen had become enormously enlarged, so much so as to resemble pregnancy at the seventh or eighth month.... Just 278 days from the date of the receipt of the wound, I delivered this young lady of a fine boy weighing eight pounds – imagine the surprise and mortification of the entire family which may be better imagined than described. Although I found the hymen intact before delivery, I gave no credence to the earnest and oft-repeated assertions of the young lady about her innocence and her purity."

Three weeks later, Dr Capers was called to see the child. The grandmother insisted "there was something wrong about the genitals". Dr Capers found a swelling in the scrotum of the baby which he immediately extracted – this swelling turned out to be a minnie bullet, battered but intact. "Picture my astonishment," says Dr Capers, "but there can be no other solution to the phenomenon." He explained the situation to the family and to his young soldier friend who "at first, most naturally, appeared skeptical, but concluded to visit the mother." Three months later, they married and later had three more children.

Egg donation

Egg donation has only been possible since IVF and GIFT have become established. In this treatment, the sperm of the male partner is used to fertilize eggs from a female donor. The embryos which are produced are transferred to the uterus of the infertile woman, where they grow normally. Unlike donor insemination, egg donation has the advantage that both partners are involved in any resulting pregnancy. Even though the infertile woman does not contribute genetically to her own child, she carries it within her own body and she gives birth to it.

What are the indications for egg donation?

Egg donation is almost exclusively used to treat women whose own ovaries are not producing any eggs. The main indication is therefore primary ovarian failure (or premature menopause). A small percentage of women stop menstruating and enter their menopause much earlier in life than normal.

In very rare cases, egg donation may also be suitable for a few other conditions. These include:
• Women whose own eggs repeatedly fail to fertilize during IVF treatments. The presumption is that there is an inherent abnormality of the eggs, which prevents fertilization. A few units are now recommending that such women consider having eggs from a donor.
• Women whose ovaries respond very badly to drug therapy to increase ovulation during IVF treatment and from whom eggs cannot be collected due to scar tissue or ovarian cyst formation. Severe endometriosis of the ovaries is one such indication. Most of these women have had extensive pelvic inflammatory disease which has severely damaged both tubes and both ovaries.
• Women without any ovarian tissue, such as those with Turner's syndrome. Turner's syndrome is a congenital disease which is caused by a woman having only one X chromosome instead of two. Turner's syndrome results in absent periods, poor breast and genital development, and shortness of stature; a few sufferers also have heart problems. All are infertile.
• Women who are carriers of severe genetic diseases which may cause their children to die or suffer greatly. These women may also request egg donation which, of course, allows them to have perfectly healthy children.

How is egg donation done?

If you are in need of donor eggs, you are probably not having menstrual cycles. This means that the lining of the uterus – the *endometrium* – is very thin and inadequate. Even if an embryo were placed there, implantation could not happen because of the inadequacy of the uterine environment. So for egg donation to be successful, it first is necessary to stimulate the uterus with hormones so that implantation can take place. Regular hormonal treatment is required to create an artificial menstrual cycle. This is done by giving the hormones oestrogen and progesterone in a cyclical fashion, usually for about three months. At the end of this time, donated eggs can be fertilized in the laboratory with the male partner's sperm, and the resulting embryos can be transferred to the artificially stimulated uterus. This actually has a very good chance of success.

Alternatively, GIFT can be done (*see* pp. 179–81). The uterus is stimulated by hormone therapy in the same way, and once an artificial menstrual cycle has been established, eggs and sperm are placed in a Fallopian tube using a laparoscope.

Egg donation treatment may actually be more difficult if you are having regular menstrual cycles, because your periods may require suppression, using various drugs, so that the embryos can be placed in the uterus at the time when they are most likely to implant. Women with Turner's syndrome are even more difficult to treat because they have had a major hormone deficiency since birth. Because they have no ovarian tissue at all, they have never made their own oestrogen. This usually results in the uterus being much less well developed than normal, and makes an embryo transfer or GIFT treatment much less likely to succeed.

What problems might I encounter?
There is, as yet, very little hard information about the problems a recipient of donor eggs may experience. It is a new field, and unlike donor insemination, which has been carried out routinely for at least 40 years, there have been only a tiny number of babies born via egg donation. The general feeling is that the problems may be rather similar to those experienced with donor insemination. However, the woman who receives a donated egg plays a much more active biological role than does the infertile man whose partner undergoes donor insemination. This may mean that egg donation will probably be attended with rather less psychological risk.

Egg donors
Egg donors are not easy to come by. Many IVF clinics use spare eggs gleaned from women undergoing IVF treatment. IVF involves

stimulating the ovaries to produce many eggs simultaneously. Most of these eggs will not be needed for the patient's treatment as, in good clinics, only two to four embryos are transferred into the uterus. The rest of the eggs are surplus to requirements. Thus, for example, if patient A produces 20 eggs during an IVF cycle, a few of these eggs would be set aside for fertilization by sperm from the male partner of patient B, who is awaiting egg donation.

All this sounds very well, but to my mind there are very severe ethical and medical drawbacks. Supposing that, of the 20 eggs obtained, 15 are reserved for patient A's own treatment and the remaining 5 are given to B? There is always the real possibility that none of the eggs allocated for A's treatment will fertilize; alternatively, none of the embryos transferred to patient A's uterus may result in a pregnancy. Meanwhile, patient B might have got pregnant with patient A's eggs. The donor is, in effect, disadvantaged by her donation, for had she received the eggs that B received, she might have become pregnant. When you consider that A may have waited a long time for the treatment, or paid a large sum for it, she clearly has had a very poor deal.

In spite of this problem, by far the more common source of donor eggs at present are patients undergoing IVF treatment. Why is this? The alternatives are very difficult. Sperm donation is physically very easy; indeed, some people would suggest that it is pleasurable. The situation is very different for egg donation. To collect eggs from an altruistic volunteer, a minor operation is needed – either laparoscopy or ultrasound needle collection through the vagina – and a general anaesthetic may be required. These procedures carry real risks, risks that are quite acceptable if a woman needs treatment but are not at all acceptable if she is gaining no possible benefit from the procedure. Indeed, many doctors would say that these risks are not ethically acceptable, under the circumstances. As if the risk of egg collection were not enough, there is the problem of ovarian stimulation. To get eggs, drug treatment with daily fertility injections is required. This also carries risks, mainly that of overstimulating the ovaries and causing cysts. Sometimes this complication requires hospital treatment. Moreover, fertility drugs require fairly intensive monitoring with daily ultrasound and blood tests – at the very least, a severe inconvenience for a working woman or one with a young family.

Some clinics try to overcome these difficulties by encouraging an infertile woman's friends or relatives to come forward to give eggs. I believe that this is fraught with danger. We have already seen why having a related sperm donor may cause innumerable problems to a child or its parents later in life. These problems are likely to be very similar for egg donation. Indeed, they may be even greater because of the amount of effort and commitment an egg donor needs to have to go through with her donation. She may well feel very possessive about any child that results and may take more than a dispassionate interest in his or her subsequent welfare and well-being.

For these reasons, clinics like mine have decided that the only logical and ethically acceptable way of obtaining donor eggs is to collect them when women come into hospital for other gynaecological procedures, such as hysterectomy or sterilization. This does not solve the ethical problems of the complications from fertility drugs, but does remove the need for a special anaesthetic or surgical procedure to collect eggs. Moreover, such women are generally strongly motivated to help others, very often having seen the suffering that infertility brings. Alternatively, they have had the pleasure of bringing up a family and want to give something to those who have not had this experience. Those coming in for sterilization also are usually quite fertile, producing eggs of good quality – hence the request for sterilization. The problem with using gynaecological patients is, however, the problem of age. Most women having sterilization or hysterectomy are close to or over 40 years old. We have already seen that, by the age of 40, most women are producing a very large proportion of abnormal eggs (*see* p. 77). It cannot be ethical to transfer defective eggs to an infertile patient, knowing that she stands a high risk of giving birth to a genetically defective baby – especially when that genetic defect has not been engendered by her own ovaries.

Telling the truth

One of the biggest criticisms of both egg and sperm donation is that they both carry more than an element of deceit. To protect their children, and to cover up what is an area of shame and guilt for many couples, there is a strong desire to keep the facts of donor conception secret from everybody, including the children.

I am certain as I can be that such secrecy is completely misguided and wrong, and that it can build huge problems for the future.

Family secrets have a habit of surfacing – usually at moments when the family is in crisis or following a severe quarrel. Imagine the consequences to children of finding out from one or other parent, in the middle of a heated quarrel or during a divorce, that they are not the offspring of their supposed fathers or mothers. A sudden rejection by, for example, a presumed father would be a very severe trauma indeed, and it may be impossible for a child to cope with this. Even in the most stable families, if the act of donor insemination is kept secret, there can be the most harmful, unforeseen circumstances.

Children conceived by donor insemination or donor eggs may be concerned to know who their genetic parents are. Most children in this situation simply want to confirm, if possible, that their genetic parents are well and healthy, but these feelings do not interfere with that of love felt for their own "adopted" family unit. This, above all, is a good reason for openness.

Not infrequently, the attitude of secrecy is endorsed or fostered by the doctors doing the procedure. A classic example is the frequent use of mixed seminal specimens. Some practitioners, in order to give a couple the illusion that a child may be genetically their own, mix the semen of the infertile male partner with that of the donor. In this way, there is always the thought that the child might just possibly be the child of its "adoptive" father, who may desire some benefit from this. I do not agree. If a couple needs the semen to be mixed, they are almost certainly not ready to consider donor insemination. To my mind, mixing semen specimens is simply compounding any problem that may arise after donor insemination. To be confused about the real parentage of one's own child is to confound the basis of family life.

PART III

Problems During Early Pregnancy

CHAPTER THIRTEEN

Early Pregnancy Loss

Miscarriage

There can be few events more distressing than a miscarriage. This burden is inevitably borne by women, but it is sometimes forgotten how difficult it can be for the man to cope with this loss. It seems particularly harsh that women who may have been trying for years to get pregnant are rather more prone to miscarriage than others. If you finally succeed in conceiving, having gone through endless investigation and years of fraught infertility treatment, a miscarriage can bring you to the point of complete despair.

We have already seen how infertile humans are. The early human embryo is very likely to fail to implant for a variety of different reasons. Some of the reasons are very obscure, and others very poorly understood by experts. If you do not know what is causing your problem, it is particularly hard to come to terms with it. Even when the embryo is implanted, early development may fail and no foetus may be formed. Worse still, late miscarriage – that is, loss of the pregnancy after the 12th week – is quite common. Here we shall look at some of the reasons for this failure, and why early embryos are apparently so ill-protected by nature.

Why is miscarriage so frequent?

We do not know what proportion of embryos normally survive and become children. Actually, the only hard evidence we have about the frequency of miscarriage is from studying patients having test-tube baby treatment (*in vitro* fertilization, or IVF). Because embryos are deliberately placed into the uterus, it is relatively easy to work out how many women have a positive pregnancy test following this, and how many miscarry or end up with a live baby. For example, when we place a single embryo into the womb after fertilizing it outside the body, there is about a 10 per cent chance of pregnancy. Unfortunately, figures from IVF treatment may not be completely reliable, because infertile women are prone to miscarry; IVF treatment itself may increase the chance of an early miscarriage.

Our solid information is therefore limited, but there is no other way of finding out precisely and accurately whether a normal woman has ovulated and, if so, whether the egg inside her body has fertilized. Knowledge from the study of natural menstrual cycles is circumstantial. We do know that, in an average month, a normal woman has a 12–20 per cent chance of getting pregnant (*see* p. 45). What we do not know is how often in her menstrual cycles she ovulates, or how often an egg becomes fertilized and, if so, how often it implants.

It has been calculated that, overall, about 23 per cent of human pregnancies are lost in the first five months. Many of these losses do occur very early, probably before the 14th day after conception, usually before a women would even know she was pregnant, because, of course, menstruation does not generally start until 14 days after ovulation. Such a very early pregnancy loss will seldom cause any symptoms.

How can you tell if you are miscarrying?

Most women who miscarry will have already felt pregnant, and usually will have had a delayed or absent period. However, a few who miscarry may be completely unaware that they were pregnant, and may not even have missed their period. Miscarriage may be heralded by one or two symptoms, or there may simply be a feeling that the pregnancy has ended.

Vaginal bleeding

This is the most common symptom, and can occur at any time after you have missed your period. Quite often bleeding commences about six weeks after the last period. It is also said that the times of greatest risk are at 8 weeks, 12 weeks and 16 weeks – that is, at the times when you would expect a period if you weren't pregnant. However, I don't believe this.

The bleeding may be quite light – not nearly as heavy as a menstrual period, or it can be very heavy indeed, with clots. On the

197

whole, the more advanced the pregnancy, the more likely you are to bleed heavily. Whatever the stage of your pregnancy, if you do have unexpected vaginal bleeding, it really is quite important to go to see your doctor immediately.

Bleeding during early pregnancy is extremely alarming and upsetting, and comes as an acute blow both to the woman and her partner. I remember when my wife had a relatively tiny amount of bleeding in early pregnancy, and I – a case-hardened gynaecologist, a miscarriage veteran – was surprised to find how very disturbed I felt. If you are in this unfortunate situation, please remember that bleeding in very early pregnancy is extremely common. We find that, in almost 50 per cent of the pregnancies we follow very closely at Hammersmith, following treatment in the infertility clinic, the women have some degree of vaginal bleeding, but very few actually abort.

The word "abort" comes as a bit of a shock to some people. An "abortion" is the medical term for any pregnancy lost before the 28th week (thereafter, it is called a "stillbirth"). This term in no way implies that the pregnancy has been interfered with. Bleeding during early pregnancy is usually called a "threatened abortion". If the bleeding becomes very heavy and it is clear that the pregnancy has definitely been lost, it is generally referred to as an "inevitable abortion". I must emphasize, though, that even very heavy bleeding does not necessarily mean that the pregnancy has definitely been lost; on occasion I have seen women bleed profusely but keep their pregnancies. One thing is reassuring: no matter how heavy the bleeding, it will not damage a pregnancy if it survives. The bleeding cannot starve the baby of nutrients or oxygen.

If you are bleeding, it will be much more obvious when you go to the toilet. Very often, woman rest in bed and the bleeding appears to stop, but as soon as they get up and walk about, and especially when they go to the toilet, they feel it all "gushing away" from them. It is natural to think that, under these circumstances, going to the toilet or walking about has, in some way, encouraged the miscarriage to worsen. This is not true. What happens is that the blood continues to seep away, collecting at the top of the vagina; on rising, this all leaks away – often in large amounts. This is not an argument against the usefulness of bedrest. It certainly has a place in preventing miscarriage as the less you exercise and move around the greater the blood flow to the pregnancy. I do think bedrest is quite sensible.

Abdominal pain

Pain in the lower part of the abdomen is extremely common in pregnancy. I must strongly emphasize that only in very few cases does it mean that you are threatening to miscarry, or, indeed, that there is anything necessarily wrong at all. None the less, crampy lower abdominal pain, especially if associated with some bleeding, strongly suggests you may be about to miscarry. The crampy pain is usually very low down and is felt in the area just around or above the pubic bone. It may also be felt in the back, or at the top of the vagina. Some women describe it rather like labour pains.

Ectopic pregnancy (*see later*) may present you with quite similar symptoms. However, with miscarriage the bleeding usually starts first and pain commences afterwards – the reverse sometimes happens in ectopic pregnancy. Whatever the situation, if you have lower abdominal cramps or severe discomfort you should contact your doctor.

Not feeling pregnant any more

Some women, having felt very pregnant (perhaps with nausea and vomiting) suddenly stop feeling the symptoms of their pregnancy. Now, before any pregnant woman reading this gets very worked up, let me stress that it is extremely common to stop feeling pregnant during a perfectly normal pregnancy. Nevertheless, it may well be worth getting an opinion from your doctor. A pregnancy test may be negative; an ultrasound scan may show lack of progress of the pregnancy.

Why do miscarriages happen?

Much of the time, the precise reason for a miscarriage is not clear. Why they are so common is a mystery. If you have been unlucky enough to miscarry repeatedly, you should certainly do your best to find a reason. The following are the more common causes.

Genetic abnormalities

An abnormal embryo is almost certainly the most common reason for miscarriage. Defective pregnancies are very common in humans; a miscarriage is really nature's safety measure for getting rid of a "bad" pregnancy as early as possible. If some of the chromosomes are abnormal, or there are too few or too many of them, an abnormal message will result in an abnormal foetus being made. At least 38 per cent of early miscarriages when carefully studied show evidence of a chromosomal defect. The most common defects responsible are:

● *Three chromosomes of one type (instead of the normal pair).* This defect is called "trisomy" and the most frequently encountered trisomy is of chromosome number 16. This is usually due to a defective egg, and is therefore much more common in older women because they are more likely to ovulate eggs which are abnormal. When an early pregnancy is examined during an ultrasound scan, trisomy is classically associated with an empty sac (the membranes in which the baby should reside) or a very much smaller baby than expected.

Studies show that if you have had one miscarriage because of a trisomy, you are more likely to have another. Moreover, if you have had a confirmed trisomic miscarriage, it might be worth considering having amniocentesis or chorion villus sampling (*see* Chapter 14) in a subsequent pregnancy, because there is a slightly increased chance of an abnormal baby going to term.

● *One X chromosome missing.* Normal girls have two X chromosomes. Occasionally one of the X chromosomes may simply be missing (so-called "monosomy"); this causes about 10–15 per cent of all miscarriages. Only about 1 per cent of pregnancies with one sex chromosome survive to birth. This defect in the few surviving children causes a condition called Turner's syndrome, which leads to deficient growth, absent periods and infertility.

● *Multiple or extra chromosomes.* This is also a common defect known as "polyploidy". The most common situation is where there is a complete extra set of chromosomes, which may be the result of an egg being fertilized by more than one sperm simultaneously. Many of these defects do not show in the baby in an early ultrasound scan, but there may be abnormalities of the placenta. Other babies show severe defects which are completely incompatible with life.

● *Changes in individual chromosomes.* These are a less common cause of miscarriage – occurring in less than 3 per cent. Some of these structural changes are inherited from one or other parent, who may carry a chromosomal abnormality even though they are perfectly "normal" individuals. The defect can be in either partner. A blood test from both partners may be helpful in these rather rare cases.

Diagnosing chromosomally defective miscarriages Unfortunately chromosome studies have to be carried out on the aborted material to be sure that there was a genetic abnormality and this has to be done on very fresh tissue, which is frequently not available. Most miscarriages are not immediately shed from the womb, but "stay put" for a few days after death has occurred. Moreover, these tests are quite unreliable if there is any trace of infection, and most of the time aborted material contains many bacteria. This is very frustrating for most couples, who dearly want to know what has caused their loss. Consequently, our knowledge about why someone has miscarried is frequently intuitive.

Gene defects A few miscarriages may rarely be caused by a gene defect. Genes are the component part of each chromosome; there are several thousand on each chromosome. Some gene defects may cause miscarriage, but most result in the much more serious problem of an abnormal baby with a disease such as cystic fibrosis or muscular dystrophy.

Hydatidiform mole

One odd cause of a miscarriage is a so-called "hydatidiform mole". This defect, which is caused by an abnormality of the chromosomes, causes a great deal of placental tissue to develop but with no foetus being formed. It is uncommon – occurring in about 1 in every 2,000 pregnancies in Britain. We know there is almost certainly an inherited tendency to produce molar pregnancy because in some communities – Malaysia, for example – it is much more common. They are also much more frequently found in older women.

Molar pregnancy often makes you feel very sick, because it produces very large amounts of the pregnancy hormone HCG. The womb is generally quite a bit larger than would be expected by the length of the pregnancy; this is because the mole expands and dilates the uterus. Hydatidiform moles are actually tumours of the placental tissue, and the tissue produced looks like many little bunches of grapes; fortunately, this kind of tumour is very seldom malignant.

I suspect that some of the old stories of numerous multiple births were, in fact, aborted molar pregnancies. The most celebrated was that of Countess Margaret, daughter of Florent IV, the Earl of Holland, who delivered on Good Friday in 1278 when she was 42 years old (moles are commoner in older women). At that one birth, she brought forth 365 infants – 182 boys, 182 girls and one hermaphrodite. They were all baptised in two large brazen dishes by the

Bishop of Treras, all the boys being called John and the girls Elizabeth. Until the last century, the dishes were on display in the village church of Losdun and were considered one of the great curiosities of Holland. Apparently (there is always a moral), the Countess had been approached by a poor woman carrying twins in her arms, asking for charity. The supplicant was insulted by the Countess, who told her that her two children were by different fathers. The poor woman is said to have cursed the Countess, praying for her to have "as many children as there are days in the year".

Moles can persist inside the womb for several weeks or even months. Your doctor may therefore want to follow you for some time after the event to make certain that you are no longer making HCG. It is very common for a small amount of residual molar tissue to take time to disappear, but usually no action is required. You may be advised to avoid getting pregnant for several months after a molar pregnancy.

Age

The age of the woman is an important factor in miscarriage. Apart from chromosome problems explained in Chapter 14, the older you are, the greater the proportion of abnormal eggs you will have in your ovaries. Such an egg can result in an embryo being formed which is not normal and not capable of becoming a proper pregnancy.

Hormonal problems

There is some evidence that you can miscarry if you are not producing the right hormones in the right amounts. Alternatively, you may be producing too much of the male hormone testosterone. In either case, the developing embryo may not implant properly.

Some women who miscarry regularly do not make enough progesterone. This is the hormone which is made by the ovary in the *corpus luteum*, after ovulation, but it is also made by the placenta (afterbirth), by which the baby attaches itself to the womb. Some doctors believe that a low blood progesterone level leads to miscarriage, but this is almost certainly untrue. If you have an abnormally low progesterone level in early pregnancy, this probably means the pregnancy is failing and not able to produce enough of this hormone. Consequently, giving extra progesterone, a very common treatment, is most unlikely to be beneficial.

Another hormonal problem that can cause miscarriage may occur if your blood level of luteinizing hormone (LH, from the pituitary gland in the brain) is abnormally high or fluctuating. Abnormalities of LH can lead to the developing egg being matured abnormally, and this may lead to a miscarriage. Abnormalities of LH hormone are common in women with polycystic ovaries.

Very rarely, other hormone problems such as thyroid abnormalities or diabetes may cause miscarriage. This is much less common than is often believed.

Abnormalities of the uterus

These are an important and relatively common problem causing miscarriage. If the womb is misshapen, perhaps because of an abnormality with which you were born (this is surprisingly common), a developing pregnancy may end with a miscarriage. Sometimes benign swellings in the uterus, such as fibroids, may make its cavity irregular, and this also may prevent a pregnancy from implanting adequately.

Congenital abnormalities, such as a double uterus, are much more likely to cause miscarriage later in pregnancy – quite often after the 12th week. They are also quite often associated with abnormalities of the cervix (when the cervix opens up prematurely – *see below*).

Adhesions inside the uterine cavity (*see* p. 91) may not only cause complete infertility but may also be associated with miscarriage.

Cervical incompetence

The cervix, or neck of the womb, is usually tightly closed, only opening a little to allow menstrual blood to escape and sperm to get in. Normally, during labour the cervix relaxes and opens wide to allow the baby in the womb to be born. However, some women have an open cervix (or "cervical incompetence" to give it its proper medical name). This may be an inborn fault or the result of a surgical injury or following a previous pregnancy. Alternatively, the muscles of the cervix may be weak, allowing the cervical canal to open as the uterus enlarges in pregnancy. This dilation of the cervix may let bacteria into the lowest part of the uterus; the infection which is caused can then inflame the membranes surrounding the baby and a miscarriage usually results.

Miscarriages caused by an open cervix usually occur quite late in pregnancy, often after the 16th week.

Intrauterine device (IUD, "coil") in place

If you get pregnant with a coil in place – a rare but distressing occurrence – there is an increased risk of miscarrying. Having said that, most pregnancies in this situation continue to term and, fortunately, there is no evidence at all that any baby will be abnormal because you have had a coil.

Environmental hazards

It is widely thought that various chemicals may cause miscarriage. One notorious example is Dioxin – you may recall the dreadful chemical factory accident in Italy which resulted in many women subsequently miscarrying their pregnancies. Wheat contaminated with lead, regrettably sent by a famine relief organization, caused some women to miscarry in Africa in the early 1980s. Some insecticides are dangerous, and intimate contact with other severe poisons in early pregnancy is probably undesirable. Certain drugs are also dangerous. The classic example is Thalidomide, the sleeping pill, which caused many miscarriages, and the birth of the children with defective limbs.

Radiation is harmful during early pregnancy. Both Hiroshima and the recent nuclear accident in the USSR at Chernobyl resulted in some women miscarrying early pregnancies. There is no evidence, however, that using a microwave oven, computer screen and word-processor in early pregnancy is harmful.

Smoking in early pregnancy is stupid if you are prone to miscarriages. There is also good evidence that marijuana (cannabis) usage can lead to loss of a pregnancy. Heavy drinking of alcohol may also cause miscarriage; chronic alcoholics tend to have more miscarriages and more abnormal children.

Infections

Several different bacteria and some viruses are thought to be responsible for very occasional miscarriages in both humans and animals. None of these germs regularly causes a problem, and exactly how rarely or commonly they cause pregnancy loss is uncertain. Your doctor will certainly screen for infection if this is indicated.

Acute and chronic illness

Very occasionally, an acute illness may cause miscarriage, usually because a high fever has damaged an early developing pregnancy.

Most common is probably severe influenza. Chronic illnesses which may occasionally cause miscarriage are high blood pressure, severe kidney disease and some rare auto-immune diseases such as lupus. With all these diseases, normal pregnancy is more usual so there is no need for great worry.

Immunological problems

There is some evidence that you can miscarry if you and your partner have similar tissue types. The developing baby is immunologically very curious. All its tissues are unique to it alone; it is quite different from its mother and yet, in spite of contact with the mother's blood supply, it is not rejected. Any other foreign tissue – for example, a kidney, skin, even bacteria – would be immediately rejected by any human with an intact immune system. It is a considerable mystery why a baby is not treated by its mother's body in the same way. For years, it was thought that the womb might be immunologically "privileged" and that foreign things in it would not be rejected; this is now clearly untrue. Some reseachers have supposed that pregnancy itself might change a mother's rejection response, but this is certainly not the whole story because tissues grafted on to pregnant women are rejected in the same way as they would be in non-pregnant individuals.

For some time, it has been thought that certain miscarriages may be caused by problems in the immune system – that is, miscarriage results from a kind of rejection response in the body of the mother. Curiously, this rejection may be more likely if mother and father have similar tissue types. Certainly, evidence in animals shows that in-breeding between close relatives can produce a much higher rate of early pregnancy loss.

If there is a degree of compatibility between male and female partners, some doctors recommend a form of immunization of the mother if she is prone to regular miscarriage. A transfusion of cells from the father is given to his partner in a relatively simple treatment. I must emphasize that I personally am extremely dubious about the value of this treatment. There are no really good figures which prove the value of this immune therapy. I am also particularly sceptical because none of the eminent doctors dishing out this therapy can explain why it should work or the precise statistical basis for their results. The history of immune therapy is full of magic cures, few of which have stood the test of time.

Abnormal blood supply or chemistry in the uterus
There is growing evidence that an abnormal blood supply in the uterus, or deficiencies in its chemistry, may be quite important as the cause of some miscarriages. Scientific work in this area is very new, but there are likely to be important developments in this area within the next few years.

Stress and psychological factors
This is very difficult to evaluate, but is important because the cause of so many miscarriages is unclear. However, women who are prone to miscarry have less risk of miscarrying again if they are looked after with tenderness and care in a subsequent pregnancy. The precise therapy that a woman receives may not actually matter; it is most interesting that simple reassurance (irrespective of any well-defined treatments) may be particularly therapeutic.

Preventing a miscarriage: general measures
Rest
The more you relax and take it easy, the better the blood flow to the baby and the more quiet your uterus will be. You should avoid getting up too early and should get to bed at a reasonable time. It is a good idea to take temporary leave from work if you can, at least until the pregnancy is firmly established, at about ten weeks or so. If you have repeated miscarriages at a particular time in a pregnancy, you should aim to take it really easy at that stage. Don't think of yourself as an invalid though – refusing to leave the house and avoiding any social life at all may make you more tense and are not likely to help.

If you have suffered many repeat miscarriages, your doctor may suggest a period of rest in the hospital. Although hospitals are hardly ever relaxing places, hospital bedrest is an option that is worth a try. Figures show that this is one of the best ways of helping women who have had several miscarriages.

Diet
A well-balanced diet may help, but you should not worry about gaining too much weight at this stage of pregnancy.

Avoiding constipation
If you have to keep straining very heavily to pass a constipated motion, you might just endanger a pregnancy which is already at risk

206

of miscarriage. For this reason, some doctors advise extra fibre in the diet (such as wholemeal bread, fruit and vegetables), and they may also suggest a little senna to keep you regular. Your doctor will advise you about which laxatives are safe.

Iron and folic acid tablets

Although people say that being short of iron makes miscarriage more likely, this is generally untrue. If you are not anaemic, iron supplements are quite unnecessary until about the 28th week.

Some clinics prescribe a small amount of folic acid. This causes no upset and is the one vitamin that is genuinely valuable if you have a tendency to miscarry.

Alcohol and smoking

A little alcohol (one or two drinks a week) is not harmful and may even help by relaxing you and quietening the uterus. Smoking has no good effect and may reduce the blood supply to the baby.

Travel

If you can avoid it, don't travel. Short, untiring journeys are fine, and gentle train journeys will do no harm. However, it is really foolish to go on long flights or skiing holidays in early pregnancy if you are prone to miscarry.

Making love

A difficult one, this! If you have regularly miscarried, it is probably sensible to avoid sex in the early pregnancy, at least until about the 12th to the 14th week. If you do suddenly feel very amorous and get carried away, don't spend the rest of the week feeling desperately guilty. The chances of miscarriage are very remote.

Sport

This is best avoided. A little gentle swimming will do no harm but avoid tennis or more strenuous sports.

Many women blame themselves for miscarrying. They feel that if only they had done less, rested more or altered their lives in some way, the loss could have been avoided. This is wrong. Although I have suggested various ways to help yourself, it can't be denied that the effect of all these measures is marginal. The truth is that it is very hard to damage a normal pregnancy, no matter what you do.

Preventing miscarriage: special treatment

Genetic causes

Tests can be done on the miscarried embryo to see if the chromo-somes are normal. Parents can also be screened by blood tests. If your blood tests are abnormal, you can get advice from your clinic about the likelihood of you having miscarriages repeatedly.

Hormonal problems

If you have a rare hormonal imbalance, it too can be detected by blood tests before pregnancy and corrected with hormone pills such as clomiphene and steroids.

Your doctor may give you progesterone after ovulation, either in the form of an injection or pessaries (which you put into the vagina at night). The treatment is controversial because many experts think that "replacement" therapy of this sort is neither effective nor necessary.

Uterine abnormalities

These can easily be detected by X-rays (hysterosalpingograms) and then treated surgically (*see* Chapter 8).

Cervical incompetence

This can be treated by a repair to your cervix before you get pregnant, or by it being stitched shut once you are. Most doctors much prefer the latter. Although this may seem like shutting the stable door a bit too late, it is the safer and more effective treatment. Stitches are put in at around 14 weeks, before cervical incompetence can cause miscarriage, and must be removed before you give birth; this does not require anaesthesia.

Coping with miscarriage

Having a miscarriage at any time is a severe shock. It is really a loss of life within you as well as an event which makes you unwell and depressed. This is much worse if you have had difficulty getting pregnant or if you have already had a miscarriage. Doctors and friends feel helpless and are only able to offer platitudes. Because doctors are trained to heal people, they find it very difficult to deal with this condition, which occurs so often in spite of treatment, and perhaps after weeks of rest, and, when it does, is so frequently inexplicable. This makes mere words sound pointless. Friends often offer clichés: "At least you didn't know the baby" or "Lucky that you've got other children". One infertile patient of mine was told by her best friend: "Don't think about it and it'll soon be all over." Such advice, though common, is remarkably unhelpful.

To make matters worse, what happens when a miscarriage occurs can be a cause for unhappiness. Apart from childbirth, miscarriage is about the most common reason for a younger woman to enter hospital. For this very reason, hospital staff unfortunately tend to treat miscarriage as routine and do not always seem as helpful as they might be. For one thing, many doctors and nurses cannot quite understand why you may feel so frightened. Very often they are perfectly kind and reassuring but don't seem to understand that you have lost a baby that was very real to you. Because the vast majority of women who miscarry go on to have a perfectly normal pregnancy within a few months, hospital staff sometimes appear a little unaware of their distress.

Having a miscarriage frequently means staying in hospital and possibly having an anaesthetic so that the remnants of the pregnancy can be removed. Frequently in the past, women who were miscarrying were admitted to obstetric units where other women were expecting a happy outcome to their pregnancies. Fortunately, things nowadays are rather better organized, even if we, as a profession, are slow to accept the severity of the trauma involved in miscarrying.

Many difficult emotions come to a head with a miscarriage. It is usual to ask yourself if you were to blame. It is rare not to be able to think of innumerable things that you might have done to yourself, which have resulted in losing your baby. This feeling is very seldom justified. Woman commonly believe that sexual activity, staying at work, stress, a sudden fall or smoking a cigarette may have brought on the miscarriage. While this kind of thinking is natural, it is very rare for any of these factors to be of any importance.

Apart from feelings of sadness and guilt, anger is a common emotion. However, there is little rational basis for this – it is seldom indeed that anybody can be said to have caused a miscarriage. Nevertheless, it is worth knowing that your unreasonable feelings of anger are a natural reaction to what seems to be an unnatural event.

I think it is essential to recognize that a miscarriage is a loss of life and not something that can be brushed away. You have been bereaved, and it is important to cry, to mourn. Some women find it helpful to see the placenta or remnants of their conception. Seeing the tissue, or the embryo, helps many come to terms with their loss. Hospital staff may be a little wary of this, but you or your partner might ask to see if this is possible.

Grieving in itself is the most important part of the healing process. You will naturally feel doubly anxious and nervous during a future pregnancy, but there are some very positive things that you can remember. The figures clearly show that even women who miscarry many, many times are likely eventually to conceive normally. You have to ask yourself how far you are prepared to try, how much trauma you are able to take. I have seen several women have normal deliveries after 10 or 12 miscarriages. Of course, if you do persist and succeed eventually, this will not wipe out your earlier distress, but it will not have been in vain.

Telling your children

Very often you will have the difficult problem of telling your children that you have lost an early pregnancy. Listen carefully to what they say and ask questions to find out what they are thinking. Show them affection, while explaining gently in a simple, direct manner what has happened to the baby; don't avoid using words like "death" or "died". There is no reason not to say why you are sad, but avoid showing that you are frightened or anxious. You must also recognize that your children may well not want to talk about things immediately, but that their questions may surface later. At all times, reassure your children that they are not the cause of what happened, and are in no danger at all. The fact that you have been away in hospital may mean that your children feel that being abandoned is a possibility in future. Many children may show quite strong signs of emotional disturbance, especially sleeplessness, anger, bed-wetting, nightmares, sudden fright or anxiety, and you should be ready to be very supportive.

Your partner

Men, too, have a very difficult time when their partner miscarries. The majority worry most about the woman's safety: "What if she bleeds to death?" is a common but unspoken question. Once your man is reassured about your state of health, he may feel sad or disappointed. Very often his grief will not be as acute as yours, and he may find it difficult to understand why you feel so deeply; this is not at all easy for him but it helps to talk together about it.

Many men also feel angry – "Why us?" is commonly asked. Others resent the need for them to be the strong or supportive partner: "I'm feeling the pain as well." Disbelief is a very common feeling, as is general sensation of pessimism – "Will we ever have a baby?" – especially if you have had difficulty in conceiving in the first place. Feelings of guilt are also frequent in men. Sometimes this may be guilt at not feeling very distressed, or even being relieved at the loss of the pregnancy. At other times, the guilt may be because he feels that he may have caused the miscarriage by making love or by not taking sufficient care of his partner in other ways. Men also need to grieve and cry, but many feel quite inhibited about this and, curiously, you as the female partner may have to be quite supportive in this situation.

Is there any hope?

If you have been infertile as a result of tubal disease or a hormonal problem, a miscarriage is proof that you can get pregnant. As a result, you should see this as a sign of real hope that you can conceive. We have analysed the figures for women who miscarry after tubal surgery or *in vitro* fertilization, and it is clear that, provided treatment is continued, the chances of a successful pregnancy are much better than 50:50. Remember that a miscarriage is sure evidence that your tubes are open, that you do ovulate and that your partner's sperm are fertile.

Trying to understand why it happened

It is natural to feel confused after a miscarriage, and it may take some time before you are ready to think of why it occurred. One of the problems is that, most of the time, the precise reason for a particular miscarriage is unknown. Hopefully, the bewildering list of causes I have given earlier will help you to ask the right questions and, if necessary, seek investigation to reduce the risk of happening again.

Ectopic Pregnancy

An ectopic pregnancy takes place when an embryo grows outside the uterine cavity. After fertilization, the egg does not manage to travel as far as the uterus, but stops on the way and it sticks and grows there. The usual place is the Fallopian tube (about 96 per cent), but

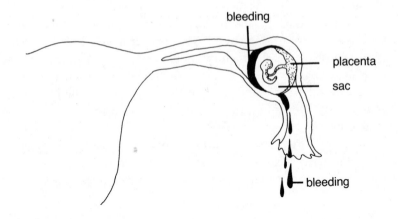

**An ectopic pregnancy in the right tube. There is some bleeding
into the tube and through the end of the tube into the tummy cavity.**

occasionally implantation happens in other places – the ovary, abdominal cavity outside the uterus or the wall of the uterus where the tube enters the uterine cavity. There is either not enough room for a pregnancy to grow properly or the placenta (afterbirth) cannot form normally. As a result, ectopic pregnancies die, or they start to bleed vigorously. This is very similar to a miscarriage, except that the bleeding is internal and occasionally can be so heavy that the situation becomes life-threatening.

Ectopic pregnancies are quite common – in the United Kingdom, at least 1 in 250 pregnancies implant outside the uterus. They are more likely with certain types of infertility (*see below*). There is also some evidence that the incidence of ectopic pregnancies is rising, possibly because so many women have damaged Fallopian tubes which predispose them to this problem.

Although having an ectopic pregnancy is an extremely upsetting event – even worse than having a miscarriage because of the pain and shock – it is worth remembering that women who have ectopics have demonstrated an ability to get pregnant. Like a miscarriage, this shows that they are ovulating, that their partner's sperm is fertile and that the eggs are capable of forming embryos. We find it most worthwhile to treat for infertility women who have previously had ectopics, as often the outlook for a successful pregnancy in the end is much better than it is for many infertile women.

What are the symptoms?
Usually there is quite a lot of pain, often to one side of the abdomen, together with light bleeding from the vagina. Quite frequently the pain is "crampy"– that is, it comes in waves. The pain generally starts before there is any bleeding. Most woman feel pregnant and normally a pregnancy test will be positive, unless the pregnancy has already started to die. If there is any internal bleeding, this can make you feel unwell – possibly sick and giddy or faint.

All these symptoms are likely to occur very early in pregnancy; you may not have even missed your period. Ectopic pregnancy is rare after about the tenth week, so if you get these symptoms later in pregnancy, they probably mean miscarriage. If you have any of these symptoms, it is vital that you contact your doctor.

Very often the diagnosis of ectopic pregnancy depends on the previous medical history (*see below*).

What causes an ectopic pregnancy?
This is not fully understood. There are several conditions that make it more likely:

● If the tube has already been damaged by infection, or is partly blocked, an ectopic pregnancy can implant in a scarred part of the tube. This is the most common reason for an ectopic.

● After embryos have been placed in the uterus during test-tube baby treatment (IVF), one of them may leave the uterus spontaneously and move into a tube, where it may implant. Such an implant is much more likely if the tubes were already damaged. Although people often believe that IVF is a way of avoiding the risk of an ectopic pregnancy, the incidence of ectopic pregnancy after IVF in women with damaged tubes is just as high as it is after tubal surgery.

● Some women who have worn an intrauterine device – an IUD or "coil" – are prone to ectopic pregnancy. This may be because the coil causes some low-grade infection. This can lead, perhaps, to damage of the cellular lining of the tube, predisposing to ectopic pregnancy.

● Woman who have already had one ectopic pregnancy are rather more likely to have another. This is because one of the tubes is invari-ably always damaged.

Diagnosis and treatment of ectopic pregnancy

The diagnosis of ectopic pregnancy can be difficult, although it has been made much easier in recent years because of the various tests that are now available. Your doctor will want to do a special pregnancy test (probably a blood test) to detect very small amounts of the pregnancy hormone HCG. Ultrasound scans can be very helpful. Nowadays vaginal ultrasound is frequently used because it gives a very accurate idea of whether there is any swelling in one or other tube. If there is any doubt about the diagnosis, laparoscopy remains the most important investigation for ectopic pregnancy.

It is not wise to leave an ectopic pregnancy inside the body once a diagnosis has been firmly made – for one thing, it can virtually never grow to a viable size. An operation is needed to remove it. Most units like to perform a laparoscopy first, and then, if an ectopic pregnancy is present, an operation is carried out to remove it.

One of the difficulties about the surgery is that the ectopic pregnancy may have damaged the tube very considerably, even if it was previously normal. As a result, most surgeons prefer to remove both the embryo and the tube it is in. While this means that you cannot have another ectopic in that tube it also means you now have only one tube to get pregnant with in future. Therefore, some surgeons try to remove the embryo alone and preserve the tube. This 'conservative' surgery is done increasingly frequently nowadays if the woman is already infertile or if there is trouble with the other tube. Although preserving the tube increases the possibility of another ectopic pregnancy (but thanks to modern techniques, the risk does not seem to be greatly increased), it does give a better chance of normal pregnancy as well.

Removal of an ectopic pregnancy usually requires an open operation which leaves a cut in the abdomen – rather similar to that used for tubal microsurgery (*see* pp. 144–7), although the surgery itself is simpler. Because ectopic pregnancies sometimes tend to bleed quite vigorously, your doctor may give you a blood transfusion. This is obviously a major operation, and it will take time to recover from it. It is quite like having your appendix removed and is not dangerous, but it means staying in hospital for about a week.

Recently there has been a vogue in some centres in the United States and France for removing ectopic pregnancies without opening the abdomen; instead, the pregnancy is sucked out of the affected tube during a laparoscopic examination. This technique is suitable if the pregnancy is quite early (and therefore small). I am very impressed with this approach, as it involves much less surgery and trauma. Unfortunately, most hospitals in the UK are, at present, unable to perform the laparoscopic removal of ectopic pregnancies. Your doctor should advise this approach only if he or she has the special expertise required and has access to the right instruments.

At present, it is not possible to take an ectopic pregnancy out of a tube and immediately replace it in the uterus. The problem is that, although the embryo may be normal, its blood supply would not regrow if this were done.

Coping with an ectopic pregnancy

Having an ectopic pregnancy is a severely traumatic experience. Many of the problems that are raised are similar to those caused by miscarriage. However, an ectopic pregnancy means a surgical procedure, which adds greatly to the upset. Unfortunately, the severity of a woman's distress is not always fully appreciated by medical and nursing staff. Because ectopic pregnancy is still largely a surgical "emergency", doctors tend to focus on the need to "save the patient's life". This anxiety is invariably communicated to relatives and friends, compounding the problem. The fact that a baby has been lost is often forgotten. Far too often, doctors are happy to say "we saved her life", neglecting the loss to the woman.

In fact, the risk involved in having an ectopic pregnancy is pretty negligible nowadays, though many patients prone to this complication live in fear of it. Modern diagnostic methods, especially laparoscopy (*see* p. 149) and ultrasound, mean that ectopic pregnancy can be diagnosed very early and that the risk of significant haemorrhage is really very small. Except in the increasingly rare cases where a Fallopian tube containing an ectopic pregnancy ruptures, causing life-treatening internal bleeding, removal of an ectopic pregnancy is certainly no more (and probably less) dangerous than having an appendix removed.

Because early diagnosis is now more common, the death of a pregnancy may be even more remote in the mind of a doctor or nurse. Early diagnosis means that tubal damage is limited; consequently, surgery may often save the tube. While it may be very reassuring to the woman to know that her tube is preserved, emphasis may be shifted away from the fact that a much-wanted baby has died.

215

What are the chances of having a second ectopic pregnancy?

If you have already had an ectopic pregnancy, you are about ten times more likely than other women to get another. Nevertheless, the odds are about 25 to 1 against, so you are still far more likely to have a normal pregnancy than to have a second ectopic. It is important to remember this, because many women become so worried about the risk of another tubal pregnancy that they use contraception indefinitely. Normal pregnancy is quite possible even after several ectopics.

> Eleni, a 30-year-old patient of mine, had had one ectopic pregnancy and her right tube had been partly removed during the operation to remove the embryo. I did some tubal surgery to repair her right tube as far as I could. She subsequently had two more ectopics, one in each tube, spaced nine months apart. Nothing daunted, she came back to see me, insisting on further tubal surgery. I told her that she was a very brave woman, but that there was no point in yet another abdominal operation. However, she eventually persuaded me to "have a go". During microsurgery I was able to repair her left tube to some extent. Since the operation she has had three babies – all girls, now aged eight, five and three. I have no idea which of her appalling-looking tubes managed to transport the embryos into the uterus.

Sometimes women find that they are unable to conceive again after an ectopic pregnancy. If this is your problem, the best thing is to have laparoscopy done to check your tubes. An ectopic often results in some adhesions forming, and it is a simple matter to check on this; you may even be able to have the problem sorted out at the same time, with the adhesions being cut during laparoscopy. Alternatively, it may be possible to repair the other tube with only a tiny risk of another ectopic. A third possibility will of course be the test-tube baby treatment (*see* Chapter 11), which has a comparatively high success rate after ectopic pregnancy.

CHAPTER FOURTEEN

Coping with Genetic Diseases

Almost certainly, the greatest worry that most pregnant women have is "Will my baby be normal?" In this chapter, I look at how efficiently we are able to detect and prevent genetic diseases before and during pregnancy, and what screening for a handicapped baby may imply for you.

It is probably no exaggeration to say that genetic disease is now the single greatest unsolved problem of modern medicine. A child born with a genetic disease will have that problem for life. Of course, a few birth defects may be surgically correctable, but when the body's chemistry is involved even surgery is unlikely to help. Many of these diseases, if not most, give rise to distressing chronic physical and mental handicap, and they are the second most common cause of babies dying at birth. In spite of the availability of screening, 1 in 50 babies are born in Britain with a major genetic defect, a typical example being spina bifida. About 1 in 100 babies have a serious or fatal disease – such as muscular dystrophy or cystic fibrosis – due to a defective gene. Most of these gene defects are inherited, but a few may occur out of the blue when there is no family background or history suggesting a particular disease. These "bolts of lightning" are so-called "gene mutations". Occasionally, in about 1 in 200 babies, there may be a problem with a whole chromosome (or part of one), which carries many genes. Such a disease is Down's syndrome.

If these gruesome statistics were not enough, it is worth considering that about 25 per cent of all children occupying a hospital bed are there because of a genetic problem. As a result, genetic disease puts a great burden on health services, as well as upon the social and educational services. Moreover, they cause difficulties and much misery for the families of affected children.

The problem of genetic disease goes further than just in children. A recent study in Britain showed that, in one average large general hospital, no less than 12 per cent of all adult in-patients were there because of a disease which was genetically related. Some genetic diseases do not surface until adulthood; others may not appear until then if they are not severe. In addition, many of the major health problems facing society have at least a genetic component – diabetes, cancer, heart attacks and much mental illness all have important contributing genetic factors.

What exactly is genetic disease?

There are two rather confusing terms. First, there is "congenital malformation". This is a defect with which a baby is born; it is occasionally, but by no means always, inherited. Second, there is "genetic defect". This is an inherited defect resulting from the action of genes.

Each cell in the body carries 23 pairs of chromosomes. One of each pair of chromosomes is inherited randomly from each parent. Each chromosome carries many hundreds of genes, each one of which is a code for a specific characteristic. Some of the characteristics produced by genes are trivial – for example, there is a gene which can give rise to blue eyes – but others are much more important because they control basic functions of the body.

Genes, which are assembled in pairs along each chromosome, are said to be *dominant* or *recessive*. If in a pair of genes one or both are dominant, this produces a recognizable effect in the body. As for recessive genes, they only produce a noticeable effect if *both* are recessive; if a recessive gene and a dominant gene are paired, the dominant gene will win. Most diseases inherited via genes are carried by recessive genes. Such recessive genes are often common, but individuals will be born with a particular disease associated with a recessive gene only if both their parents carried that particular gene and both passed it on to their child. An exception to this general rule is if an individual is born with a mutant gene, arising anew as a result of fresh chemical action. He or she may be affected with a particular genetic disease, even though the parents were not genetic carriers.

A genetic disorder can be one of four different types.

Single gene defects

The number of diseases caused by single defective genes is, curiously, not precisely known, although it is estimated that there are about 3,370 of them. Roughly one-half of these are caused by dominant genes, rather fewer by recessive genes and the remainder are sex linked – that is, they are carried on the X chromosome and their inheritance depends on the sex of the baby.

Dominant genetic disease

Most diseases caused by dominant genes are rare. This is because, if the gene is present, the offspring will have the disease and die before being able to reproduce. The exceptions are if the dominant gene does not produce a fatal disease, or if the disease is not severe enough to prevent a sexual relationship or pregnancy. The most common dominant genetic disease is probably hypercholesterolaemia – an abnormally high level of cholesterol in the blood which leads to early death in young adults (in their 20s and onwards) from heart attacks. This occurs in 1 in 500 births. Another well-known disease is Huntington's chorea, occurring in 1 in 2,000 births, causing loss of muscle control, dementia and death in middle age. This is a terrifying disease to have in the family, because members of the family, who have intimate knowledge of its appalling consequences, have to wait to find out whether they also have this dominant gene. If they do, they will start to experience themselves the horrifying deterioration that they have previously witnessed in a loved one.

Recessive genetic disease

The most common recessive genetic disease is cystic fibrosis, carried by 1 in 20 of the population. Because both parents need to have a recessive gene for their children to have the actual disease, 1 in 400 couples (20 × 20) are at risk of having a child with this illness. Cystic fibrosis causes deficient digestion and recurrent chest infections. This does not sound so bad, but the disease usually requires multiple hospital admissions and daily treatments, and the majority of sufferers die in childhood, though a few survive (usually very disabled) into young adult life. Apart from the hardship to the sufferers and their families, it has been estimated that it costs up to £15,000 annually to keep a child with this illness alive.

Some recessive genetic diseases are much more common in certain parts of the world or in certain racial (and interrelated) groups.

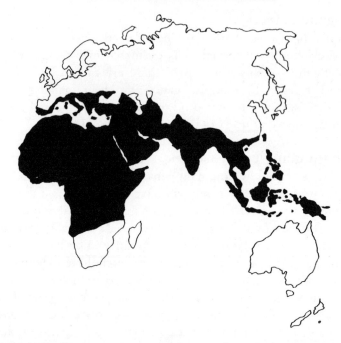

Countries (shaded in black) where people are most likely to inherit the blood disease, ß-thalassaemia.

Thalassaemia, a very serious blood disease causing severe disability, is a typical example. Although it only occurs in 1 in 20,000 births in the general population, it is very common in people of Mediterranean origin. For example 1 in 50 babies born to Cypriots living in London suffers from this terrible illness. At least 200,000 babies are born annually around the world with this disease – in Thailand alone, there are thought to be some 500,000 children suffering from some form of thalassaemia. Most of these, in spite of inadequate but expensive treatment – will die by the age of 5.

Sex-linked disease

The sex-linked diseases are usually passed on by females but only boys are affected. The most important of these is Duchenne muscular dystrophy, which causes progressive muscular weakness. One in 5,000 boys born in Britain suffer from it. These children are usually confined to wheelchairs; death occurs when they can no longer use

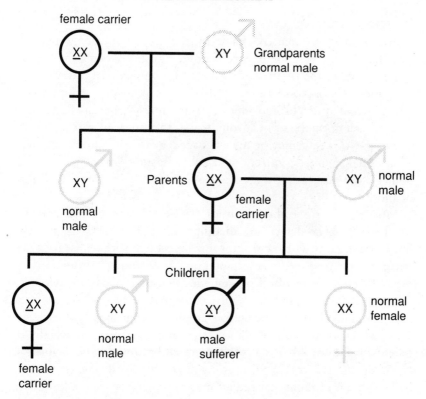

female carrier

XX

XY Grandparents
normal male

XY

normal
male

Parents XX

female
carrier

XY normal
male

Children

XX

female
carrier

XY

normal
male

XY

male
sufferer

XX normal
female

**The family tree of a typical family with haemophilia. This is a
sex-linked gene carried on the X chromosome by females; 50 per
cent of their male children will be affected and 50 per cent of the
daughters will be carriers. In a family with four children, on
average two will be boys, and one affected.**

their breathing muscles. A disease that is more well known (though
less common) is haemophilia – it has attracted popular attention
because this was the notorious disease that afflicted the unfortunate
Russian royal family and was carried by Queen Victoria. The blood
of haemophiliacs does not clot properly, and they are therefore in
danger of uncontrolled bleeding. This can be avoided if they take
Factor VIII, a component of blood.

Chromosome defects

Chromosomes are paired. Each of the 23 chromosome pairs is classified according to size, chromosome pair no. 1 being the biggest and pair no. 22 the smallest. Pair no. 23 is composed of the sex chromosomes, XX or XY. Diseases caused by chromosome defects occur when one or more chromosomes carrying many genes are abnormal. Instead of a normal pair of chromosomes there may be three; alternatively, one of a pair may be missing (*see* Turner's syndrome, p. 190). Occasionally only a piece of a chromosome may be missing. Sometimes, one chromosome from one pair may be mixed with that of another.

Most chromosome abnormalities, because they involve several and not just one gene defect, are incompatible with life. Consequently, most pregnancies with a chromosome defect end with a miscarriage – nature's "safety valve" (*see* Chapter 13). It seems extraordinary that, over all, 15 per cent of all pregnancies that end in a birth involve a chromosome defect, that is about 1 in 190 babies. When you consider how common chromosome defects are, it is astonishing how little we know about the causes. We know that abnormal eggs, especially in older women, are likely to result in an embryo with three copies of chromosome 21 – this in turn results in Down's syndrome (*see* p. 77). Although it is thought that radiation, some chemicals and a few other environmental factors may cause some chromosome defects, the cause of most is entirely unclear. This remains a major area for research.

Congenital malformations

Some congenital malformations have a genetic origin. When they do, it is usually because several genes are acting together. Consequently, their inheritance does not follow any precise pattern, but people who have given birth to a baby with certain genetic defects may have a high chance of conceiving another affected child – probably a risk of about 1 in 20. An example of a very common disease with a strong genetic component is spina bifida, a "neural tube defect" in which part of the spinal cord bulges out of a gap in the backbone. These children with this disorder may, if they survive, be confined to a wheelchair and have defective bladder and bowel function.

Not all congenital malformations are genetic. Some are due to viruses. Others may be due to exposure to radiation, vitamin deficiency, chemicals or drugs. An example of the latter is, of course, Thalidomide. It is most important to recognize that most malformations occur as a matter of pure chance. Far too frequently, people blame themselves for what has happened to their children.

Illnesses with a genetic component

These illnesses are indeed numerous. Diabetes, which occurs in about 0.5 per cent of the population, is one. Schizophrenia, affecting 1 per cent, is another. The list is extensive, and includes coronary heart disease, arthritis, multiple sclerosis, certain types of infertility (especially those associated with defects of the ovary or uterus), some forms of mental retardation, and some of the rarer types of cancer. All these illnesses are probably caused, at least in part, by several genes acting together in the body.

Preventing genetic disease

Only a minority of genetic diseases can be effectively treated. Consequently, prevention remains the biggest weapon we have in fighting genetic diseases. It can be accomplished in two ways. Using modern methods of chemical or DNA analysis (DNA being the material from which chromosomes are made), couples can be screened before conceiving and then counselled. Unfortunately, this type of screening is presently only possible for very few diseases. Moreover, because these diseases usually arise from two parents with the same recessive gene, the best prevention that can be achieved is by advising such couples not to have children. The other method of prevention involves identifying couples at risk, and offering to terminate any pregnancy which may be affected.

Neither of these is satisfactory. Genetic counselling is obviously limited because there are few diseases we can identify in prospective parents. On the other hand, termination of pregnancy is fraught with all sorts of ethical and emotional problems. Apart from any moral arguments against killing a foetus, so-called "therapeutic abortion" has harsh implications for the mother. The effect that terminating a pregnancy has on women (and indeed men) has been trivialized by our society. Apart from medical complications, which are not that infrequent, many if not most women feel very sad and are often profoundly depressed following termination. These feelings can be much deeper than is often supposed and some couples feel permanent grief at the deliberate termination of a pregnancy. Apart from any religious considerations, this, I believe, is why there has been a growing realization that bringing up a handicapped child may be a preferable option for some couples.

Antenatal diagnosis
Amniocentesis

Many genetic defects can be diagnosed in time to consider termination of the pregnancy and amniocentesis is the most common diagnostic method. It involves taking some fluid from the sac surrounding the baby. The cells from the baby can be analysed as well as any chemicals it excretes.

Most chromosomal defects can be identified reasonably reliably by this method. Many other defects which involve abnormal body chemistry can also be detected, provided, of course, that the doctors know for which chemicals to test; an example is Tay-Sachs disease (which causes babies to die from progressive brain deterioration by the age of 2). Amniocentesis is a very safe procedure in good hands, carrying only perhaps a 1 in 200 chance of starting a miscarriage.

The disadvantages of amniocentesis are that the sac surrounding the baby is usually not big enough for safe sampling until about the 15th or 16th week of pregnancy. Moreover, because there are only very few cells floating in the amniotic fluid, they have to be grown in a culture before a chromosome test can be done reliably; this may take three weeks or more. If there is a chromosomal defect, the pregnancy may be very advanced – perhaps 19 weeks at the earliest – before a decision to terminate can be made. This can be very traumatic because, by this time, the baby can be felt moving and there is inevitably a commitment to being pregnant. Moreover, termination involves going through a form of labour, which is obviously very unpleasant.

Chorion villus sampling

Recently, another method for antenatal diagnosis has been developed. Chorion villus sampling – called CVS for short – involves taking a small piece from the baby's side of the placenta away for analysis. Because both the baby and its placental tissue derive from the same cells, cells from the placenta accurately reflect the condition of the baby. CVS can be done either by sucking a few placental cells away through a tube inserted through the cervix, or by inserting a needle through the woman's abdominal wall. With the latter technique (and sometimes the former), ultrasound is used to guide the doctor so that the baby and its membranes are left undamaged.

Chorion villus sampling can be done much earlier in pregnancy than amniocentesis, usually between 9 and 11 weeks. Moreover, diagnosis of many defects is fairly rapid, particularly when a specific gene defect is suspected. Modern methods of DNA analysis mean that a diagnosis should not take longer than two weeks; indeed, using a new method called *polymerase chain reaction* (PCR), many gene defects can be diagnosed within 24 hours. The advantages are considerable, because termination of an early pregnancy is much less traumatic. Also, if PCR can be used, the emotional stress of waiting for a diagnosis is substantially reduced. Chorion villus sampling can also be used for testing for chromosome abnormalities, but a firm diagnosis of this may often take up to two weeks. The main disadvantage of CVS is that it carries a slightly greater risk of miscarriage than amniocentesis – around 1 per cent.

There have now been well over 60,000 CVS samples done around the world. These are recorded in a central data register in Philadelphia, and there has been no evidence of any risk of this technique causing an abnormal baby. Unfortunately, in the event of a doubtful CVS result (particularly with some chromosomal problems), amniocentesis may be very occasionally required at a later date to confirm that the baby is normal.

Other techniques of antenatal diagnosis

There are other important methods for detecting defects, which should be mentioned to complete the picture.

Ultrasound. Ultrasonic examination of babies is now, of course, commonplace. It clearly ranks as one of the greatest advances in modern obstetrics for helping doctors to follow accurately the progress of a baby's growth in the womb. All available evidence shows that this is an extremely safe method.

In recent years, ultrasound has become even more accurate and the pictures through it have a better resolution. This means that a better view of the baby can be obtained and certain foetal defects can be diagnosed with it. Perhaps the three which are most important in earlier pregnancies are defects of the spinal cord, certain abnormalities of the head and defects of the heart. Unfortunately, even these are difficult to diagnose before about 18–19 weeks, which is very late to consider terminating pregnancy. Moreover, accurate diagnosis depends a good deal upon the operator's experience and in any case, not all routine ultrasound examinations, will, pick up all such defects, especially if they are small.

Chordocentesis. (foetal blood sampling) It is now actually possible to take blood from the baby in the womb. This is done by chordocentesis: after an injection of a little local anaesthetic is given, a needle is guided painlessly through the woman's abdominal wall into the womb and then into the baby's umbilical cord. Ultrasound is required to guide the needle. This test can be done from 17 weeks onwards. It requires special skill, but is safe, carrying no greater risk of miscarriage than CVS – i.e. about 1 per cent. It has the advantage over amniocentesis in that actual blood cells are retrieved, which can lead to a rapid diagnosis of chromosome problems. Usually an answer can be obtained within a few days of the test.

Foetoscopy. Some specialists in antenatal diagnosis insert a special telescope (known as a foetoscope), no thicker than a ball-point pen refill, into the uterus, to look at the baby. Certain rare liver and skin diseases in the baby can be diagnosed this way. The examination is painless, though a little local anaesthetic is needed in the skin of the woman's abdomen.

Maternal blood tests. It has been known for quite a time that the babies of women with raised levels of a chemical called alphafoetoprotein (AFP) are more likely to have spinal cord defects such as spina bifida. This can be reliably detected in the fluid surrounding the baby after amniocentesis at around 12–14 weeks. AFP is also slightly raised in the woman's bloodstream in such pregnancies. However, the rise is small and blood tests alone are not reliable; amniocentesis must be done to confirm the diagnosis.

There has recently been a dramatic new use found for AFP blood testing. A team at St Bartholomew's Hospital in London has found that women carrying babies with Down's syndrome are more likely to have a lower-than-normal blood level of AFP as well as raised blood levels of HCG and a hormone called estriol. They found that if they tested levels of all three at once, they had a rapid screening test for Down's syndrome, which could be done at around 16 weeks. This is important. At present in Britain, only about 15 per cent of all Down's syndrome babies are detected before birth. This screening test, if widely done in pregnancy, would certainly lead to more women at high risk subsequently going on to have amniocentesis and to the detection of at least 70 per cent of cases of Down's syndrome.

An abnormal baby: choosing what to do

Once an abnormal baby has been detected, parents have a hard decision to make. Abortion is now widely accepted by our society, but is certainly not the right choice for everybody. Many people, particularly those who are deeply religious, believe that abortion is not a choice at all, and they will rightly refuse screening by amniocentesis or CVS.

However, it is not only those with deeply held religious views who do not accept abortion; some people simply feel that the baby has a right to life and that it is morally wrong to tamper with any pregnancy. They frequently point out that although there may be physical or mental impairment, many of these defects are quite compatible with a happy life. Children with Down's syndrome are an excellent example: given a stimulating environment, these children, who tend naturally to be happy, often develop remarkably well.

There is also no doubt that many women will refuse amniocentesis because of its lateness. As one woman said to me, "I would have liked CVS earlier in this pregnancy had it been available, but I feel unable to go through amniocentesis now with this feeling that I would be destroying my living, moving child." Another reason for refusing amniocentesis is the risk, however small, of miscarriage. Some women feel that they cannot accept even the remotest risk of damaging a normal baby.

Of course, the great majority of women who find that their babies are abnormal decide to terminate their pregnancies. This is partly because most of those who undergo ante-natal testing have already made this decision if they are found to have a baby with a foetal abnormality. In spite of this, many women find that they are having to make a fresh decision when actually faced with the bad news. It may be an easier decision to make when the baby has a fatal condition, though there will still be feelings of guilt and deep responsibility. These feelings are heightened for most women when they are told that their babies have an abnormality such as Down's syndrome, because they recognize that such a baby may live to quite an advanced age.

Whatever the decision is, grief is an important process which needs to be gone through. Fortunately, clinics now are more supportive and many have sensible counselling services, though often these still fall well short of ideal.

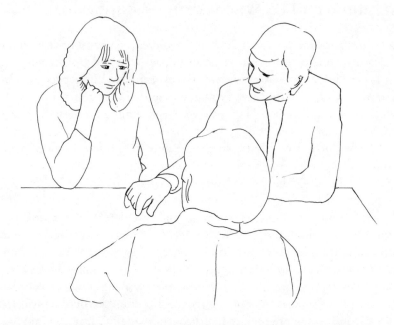

If an abnormality is detected, parents will have to make a big decision about the future. The doctor will explain what has happened and what are the options.

Getting the test result

Finding out that your baby is abnormal is a horrible, numbing shock. The mutual support of both partners can be very important when you get the news and also when you have to make decisions. In my view, the man should always be encouraged to be with the woman during the amniocentesis or ultrasound examination, and certainly when returning to the antenatal clinic to get test results. Unfortunately (and, I think, wrongly), some women are given these results by telephone. I think it better that they should be handled face to face, with the doctor and both partners present. Male partners should also, in my opinion, recognize that they will be needed much more at home following a "bad" diagnosis.

Although sharing the grief may be important, men and women react differently to termination. The experience itself cannot be entirely shared – after all, the baby grows and moves inside the woman, not the man. Of course the knowledge of a defective baby

228

can draw some couples closer together. However, no matter how shocked they are, men usually find it easier to cope with a termination, for example, immersing themselves in their work. Most women take longer in their grieving, not least because of the physical changes that a pregnancy has demanded of their bodies. The fact that a woman may still be mourning while her partner is apparently remote can drive a couple apart. It may also be very important for a woman to find other people in whom she can confide, perhaps a close friend or relative. This may also be extremely helpful when deciding whether to terminate or not.

The medical profession has not been very good in this situation. Up to now, there has been remarkably little support for couples taking these momentous decisions, for the bereaved couple who have undergone a termination, or the couple who have decided to keep a damaged child. There is no doubt that parents, especially women, are put under huge pressure by our society, which finds it difficult to accept, understand or tolerate handicap. There is an assumption that a couple, and especially the woman, will rapidly "get over it". Some doctors and nurses are even insensitive enough to imply that "another pregnancy" will soon make a couple forget the unhappiness of this one. Such attitudes are becoming less common, and fortunately, there is the slowly growing recognition that people need much more support and counselling.

There is also too little sensitively written information. Too much has been published that contains only medical facts and easy solutions (usually written, I fear, by doctors). Alternatively, there are one or two very angry books which are virulently feminist – these, I think, would be damaging and disturbing for most women facing these questions. One book I strongly recommend is *The Tentative Pregnancy* by Barbara Katz Rothman. This offers sensitive and compassionate advice to women considering whether to undergo amniocentesis and termination of pregnancy.

CHAPTER FIFTEEN

Research: Ethics and Popular Attitudes

The treatment of infertility and research into human reproduction raises many questions of particular interest to those who are trying to have children. Some of the ethical matters are beyond the scope of this book, but the key issue of research on human embryos is especially relevant as well as of wide interest and great importance. Few reproductive scientists doubt that embryo research offers answers to many of the questions raised in this book.

The case for embryo research

Infertility

There is no doubt that research with human embryos is crucial if we are to improve the comparatively poor results of infertility treatment. *In vitro* fertilization itself would not have been possible without embryo research. Human embryos had to be studied after fertilization outside the body to ensure that such an artificial environment does not cause any birth defects. Regrettably, IVF remains one of the least successful of all fertility treatments. We do not understand, for example, why the culture conditions we use in the laboratory result in only about 10 per cent of healthy-looking embryos successfully implanting after transfer to the uterus. Treatment of male infertility is even more unreliable. We saw in Chapter 9 that only about 10 per cent of infertile men have a treatable defect. New treatments, such as sperm injection into the egg (*see* p. 170), require the scientist to ensure that embryos generated by such

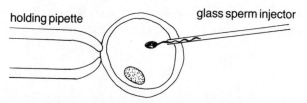

(1) Sperm injection for male infertility

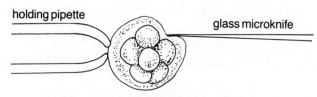

(2) Embryo biopsy for genetic diagnosis

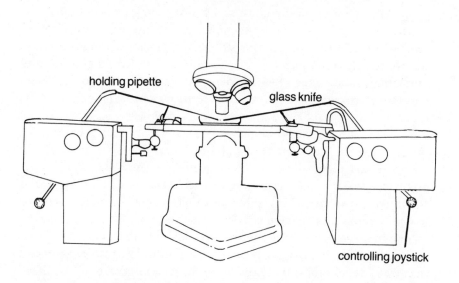

Micromanipulation. This may potentially be for injecting the sperm into the egg in some case of male infertility, or to remove one cell from an embryo to diagnose a genetic disease. These techniques are still experimental. The microscope set up with glass biopsy knives held either side in micromanipulators. (1) Sperm injection. The egg is held by a glass holding pipette using gentle suction; sperm injection is done with a very fine glass tube. (2) A six- or eight-cell embryo has one cell removed through a minute hole made by a glass microknife. This cell will then be subjected to chemical analysis.

methods are normal, and cannot give rise to damaged babies. Such work, though started in animals, must be completed using human embryos because animals do not suffer the same birth defects.

Genetic disease

Embryo research is also vital if we are to improve our understanding and handling of genetic diseases. I have already indicated that these represent one of the greatest unsolved problems in modern medicine. Many, if not most, of these diseases are unique to humans and cannot be tackled or properly investigated using animal eggs and sperm. Although some research can be done looking at other cells in culture, it is the early embryo which goes wrong, and it is this which requires closest study.

A very good example of the value of embryo research is the recent advance of pre-implantation diagnosis. In the previous chapter, we saw that CVS is generally more acceptable than amniocentesis in the antenatal diagnosis of abnormal babies, because this can occur so much earlier. Nevertheless, this still leaves a couple facing a decision regarding termination. A very recent breakthrough is pre-implantation diagnosis – the diagnosis of an embryonic defect between two and five days after fertilization. More research is needed, but it is likely that, very soon, couples at known risk of producing a genetically damaged baby will be able to start a pregnancy reassured that their baby is free of that specific defect. In Chapter 4, I mentioned that new technology will almost certainly allow the selection of a baby's sex, where there is a known risk of a sex-linked disorder. This same technology will also be used for couples who carry specific gene defects, and possibly for some who are at greater than average risk of a chromosome defect.

Pre-implantation diagnosis presently requires IVF. No pregnancies have yet been established after a pre-implantation diagnosis has been made, but this is likely to happen soon. The procedure will be that the woman will be stimulated with fertility drugs to produce several eggs simultaneously; these will be fertilized by her partner's semen. About three days after fertilization, a single cell can be removed from each embryo. These cells would be examined for the specific gene defect, using methods such as PCR (*see* p. 225) for analysing the DNA. This can be done extremely rapidly, and it should then be possible to transfer only normal embryos to the mother's womb by the evening of the third day after fertilization. This is well before the embryo would normally implant; indeed, it is before a woman could possibly know she might be pregnant – around the 18th day of her menstrual cycle. The emotional advantages of such an approach are overwhelming. Moreover, the technique overcomes the religious problems and moral qualms that many couples feel over termination of pregnancy.

> Sheila knew that she might be a carrier of a genetic disease only after she had watched her 14-year-old brother die from muscular dystrophy. He had spent the last six years of his life increasingly incapacitated, in a wheelchair. Sheila's blood test suggested that she might be a genetic carrier of the disease, which meant that any of her own sons could suffer a similar fate.
>
> Sheila married at 19. Her first two pregnancies were tested, found to be affected and were terminated at 22 weeks of pregnancy. Her husband could not cope with this, nor with Sheila's sadness and remorse. Their marriage broke up.
>
> Since then Sheila has remarried and has had three more pregnancies. All three babies were diagnosed as having the disease and all have been aborted. Now neither she nor John, her husband, feel they can embark on another pregnancy and face the desolation of another termination. Both desperately want children. Pre-implantation diagnosis would be a great benefit to them.

There are, however, two problems with pre-implantation diagnosis which still require careful investigation. The first is whether, by taking a cell away for examination from a human embryo, scientists might actually cause a defect. The second is whether examination of a single cell from the embryo is really representative and also reliable. Both of these problems require careful research using human embryos. Unfortunately, there has been a huge campaign conducted against embryo research. This has delayed important, valuable scientific advances because units have been reluctant to invest hard-pressed funds and academic energy into an area which might be prematurely banned by hasty legislation.

Miscarriage

A third reason for embryo research is the problem of miscarriage. In Britain alone, over 100,000 women each year are admitted to hospital with threatened or incomplete miscarriages. Leaving aside the huge financial cost, there is a huge emotional cost which even doctors are only just beginning to understand. A miscarriage also involves considerable health risks and quite a few women remain infertile afterwards; others may develop painful symptoms of chronic pelvic infection.

In 80 per cent of cases, we have very little idea what really has caused a miscarriage. We know that most miscarried pregnancies arise from abnormal embryos, but we have very little idea of what causes those abnormal embryos in the first place, and what measures might prevent those abnormalities. There can be little doubt that human embryo research is essential if we are to make any serious progress in this field.

Implantation and ectopic pregnancy

A fourth reason for embryo research is to understand how embryos implant. We know that the majority of human embryos actually fail to implant in the womb, and are lost. Some are abnormal, of course, but by no means all. If we knew how human embryos implant, and what chemical messages pass between the embryo and womb, we would be in a better position to understand miscarriage, contraception, ectopic pregnancy and early development. Ectopic pregnancy is a dangerous emergency. In Jamaica, about 1 in 15 pregnancies are ectopic; ectopics, especially in countries with limited health care, are one of the most common causes of women dying in pregnancy. Yet ectopic pregnancy (*see* Chapter 13) is a mystifying condition; we simply do not know why so many pregnancies implant inside the tube. Ectopic pregnancy is virtually unknown in any animal species apart from man. There seems to be something peculiar about human implantation which predisposes women to this important problem.

Cancer

It may seem extraordinary to suggest that embryo research could give insights into the understanding and treatment of cancer. None the less, several researchers are pursuing investigations in this area. Every cell in the body carries a group of genes called *oncogenes* – the "housekeeping" genes that control each cell's growth and division. Cancer is basically a disease in which some cells start to divide very rapidly and abnormally. If we knew what goes wrong with the genes controlling cell division, we might have sufficient insight to work out new treatments. The early embryonic cells, which provide an ideal model for the action of oncogenes, are in many ways perfect for this kind of study.

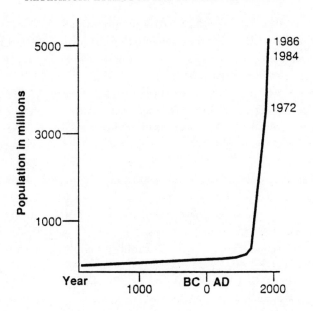

The burgeoning population of the world.

Contraception

Another problem is the world's burgeoning population. The graph dramatically shows the scope of the problem. Although the population of the world has grown frighteningly, most estimates suggest that the rate of growth may now be slowing. Nevertheless, the United Nations estimates that, by the year 2100, it will reach 10,185 million – twice what it is now. Other estimates put it at considerably more than this. Whatever the speed of growth, it is clear that the populations of Europe and North America will remain relatively static, and that the main burden of this huge increase in humanity will be borne by the poorest nations who can least afford to support it. It is this threat, above all, which has stimulated the World Health Organization's attempts to improve existing methods of contraception.

Most current methods of contraception are short of ideal. Most have side-effects and some have potential dangers. Sterilization, both male and female, is largely irreversible and therefore often unacceptable. A new approach is needed. Work is in progress to look at methods of immunizing people against an early developing pregnancy. Other alternatives are substances which interfere with fertilization or with early embryonic growth. Embryo research is vital in the investigation of all of these different methods, not least because it will be essential to ensure that such methods do not cause damage to an embryo which "slips through the contraceptive net", in the event of contraceptive failure. While an occasional failure of a contraceptive method is just acceptable, this would not be so if a deformed or damaged baby was born as a result of contraceptive usage.

To be fair, my graph may be too gloomy. Incorrect predictions of catastrophe are not new. In 1798, Thomas Malthus calculated that Britain's population would rise from its then 7 million to 112 million by 1900. He also thought that, by 1900, food supplies in Britain would support no more than 35 million people, and he forecast famine or enforced mass emigration. However, there was no solution to his perceived dilemma as the population in the rest of the world would have expanded in a similar way, which would not have helped emigrés. We know now that Malthus was wrong. Even without contraception, British population growth did not meet his worst expectations but slowed substantially. The factors which brought this about were largely social. There were great improvements in living standards, in diet, in social equality, in education and in political and social stability. The death rate decreased with improvements in health care and the prevention of disease. All this led to what has been termed "population maturation" with a fall in birth rate in developed countries: people no longer felt the need to have large families because so many more of their children were surviving.

Things are different in developing countries. While the introduction of Western-style medicine has caused death rates to fall rapidly and dramatically, the birth rate remains high. The difference is that, in the West, the death rate came down gradually over 200 years, and the birth rate responded by falling approximately 50 years later. In developing countries, the drop in the death rate has been too sudden and rapid for us to expect to see a corresponding fall in birth rate. Moreover, most developing countries remain pitifully poor and relatively unstable. Consequently, we are yet to witness the effect of population maturation in the developing world.

It is a horrifying paradox to consider how Western medicine and attitudes have, in certain ways, caused very difficult problems in the developing world. A few years ago, I was in a children's care centre in rural India. There were perhaps 300 orphans standing around in a primitive playing field, all between the ages of 5 and 7; none was the size of my own 4-year-old child. It suddenly occurred to me that, were vaccination and antibiotics not available, few of these children would be alive.

One natural method of contraception is breastfeeding. While a woman is lactating, her periods stop and she seldom ovulates. Women of the Kung tribe from the Kalahari, who marry very young yet use no form of contraception nor abortion, breastfeed their babies by continuous suckling for at least three years after birth. This provides an ideal way of limiting family size and they have an average of fewer than five babies per family. You may remember Mrs McNaught who I mentioned in Chapter 1. She gave birth, in separate pregnancies, to 12 boys and 10 girls in 28 years. After each pregnancy, her doctor gave her injections to stop her breast milk. Perhaps if she had breastfed her babies, she might not be in the *Guinness Book of Records*.

WHO point out that we should encourage far more breastfeeding, especially in developing countries. Cow's milk or powdered substitutes, given in bottles, are a potent cause of serious disease and fatal diarrhoea in hot countries, where infections cannot be controlled. Pope John Paul II, in his *Humanæ Vitæ*, has insisted that contraception is wrong except where "natural cycles" are used. This causes great difficulties for the 800 million Catholics in the world. The Church could do much by encouraging breastfeeding. Less insistence on sexual abstinence and more emphasis on lactation might cut birth rates and ensure fewer infant deaths from gastro-enteritis and similar causes.

The case against embryo research

Opposition to embryo research is based partly on moral or religious grounds and partly on the fear of a misuse of technology. Many arguments have been put forward.

"Human life begins at conception and is sacrosanct."

This is the most potent of religious arguments. It takes various forms: that the human embryo is a person or that it is "human" and, as such, is entitled to be protected like any other human. This argument

"The slippery slope"

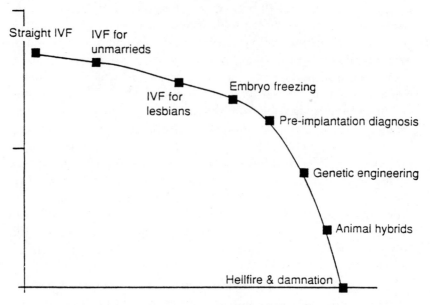

Straight IVF IVF for unmarrieds · IVF for lesbians · Embryo freezing · Pre-implantation diagnosis · Genetic engineering · Animal hybrids · Hellfire & damnation

eventually comes down to a matter of belief. I personally find it difficult to accept that the embryo, a mere ball of undifferentiated cells with only limited potential for development, can be equated with a foetus – which has organs and which moves and which at least has a better than even chance of survival in the womb. It seems to me that our society, by the widespread use of contraceptive preparations which lead to embryonic destruction has already decided the status of the human embryo. Moreover, if human life begins at conception, is the egg or the sperm not "human" or not alive? And, bearing in mind that fertilization is a lengthy process, if life begins at conception, at which precise moment is that?

"The human embryo is a unique individual."

This statement depends on the fact that each embryo has its own unique set of genes, which will give rise to its own unique attributes should it implant successfully. This argument is easier to refute. We know that twins can be formed at seven days after fertilization and, occasionally, as late as 14 days. Identical twins are formed when the "unique " embryo splits into two. Of course, "uniqueness" is not only a property of the embryo; as we have seen, each egg and each sperm are also unique.

"No good has come from embryo research."

Strangely, this argument has been heard frequently and in every debate on the subject. It is simply untrue. Without embryo research, *in vitro* fertilization would not have been developed. Moreover, we have also seen how embryo research is now helping in the battle against genetic disease.

"A time limit is the start of a slippery slope."

A common argument is that if society allows scientists to experiment up to a certain number of days after fertilization (14 days in Britain), scientists will want to extend this period if it becomes expedient or useful to do so. To my mind, this argument is fallacious. The medical profession already has many limits imposed on it concerning what is ethical in research, and these limits are fully and totally accepted. A variation of the argument is that if scientists are allowed to experiment on embryos, they will not stop at a point that is generally acceptable.

"Embryo research is a licence for genetic engineering."

Very many people are concerned that embryo research will be used to create human beings with "desirable" characteristics. Genetic engineering, it is widely believed, could be misused to produce super-intelligent or very aggressive beings who would be modelled by politicians to subjugate others. There are many variations on this theme. The idea of producing a Hitler clone (along the lines of Ira Levin's novel *The Boys from Brazil*), for example, is one that rightly horrifies very many people.

Scientists universally agree that genetic engineering of "desirable" characteristics is likely to be unpredictable, if not impossible. Such characteristics are produced by the multiple action of many genes, which would seem to be an insurmountable problem even if anyone wished to do such work (which they do not). It would be much simpler to manipulate the education and environment to produce a "master race". Moreover, there has been universal agreement among all scientists that any form of tampering with human genetic structure is completely unacceptable. Nevertheless, open regulation by government inspection and policing would serve the interests of society better than to risk secret experimentation of a banned technology.

239

"People who are infertile have brought it upon themselves."

The implication is that research into infertility is not worthwhile, because infertile people have created their own problem by carelessness or promiscuous behaviour. The argument runs along the lines of "Why get into grey moral areas for the sake of people who are not worthy?" This remarkably callous and unfair argument was presented by more than one politician during debates on embryo research.

"Any research that is needed can be done using animals."

Animal research is most important in understanding human reproduction; indeed, it is vital that animal research continue. Unfortunately, study of animal embryos is no substitute for human research. Animals do not suffer the same genetic diseases as humans, they have different genes and chromosomes, rarely have miscarriages, virtually never suffer ectopic pregnancy, and are, in general, far more fertile.

"The campaign against embryo research."

Although research into human reproduction and IVF is not particularly new (Dr Robert Edwards was doing his studies on human embryos over 15 years ago), the campaign to stop embryo research is recent. There was growing awareness in the early 1980s that IVF technology involved the generation of surplus embryos. It was also realized that genetic manipulation, cloning, animal hybrids and human embryo storage were matters of public concern.

The Warnock Committee was established by the British government to look into these and related areas. Having taken copious evidence over two years, the Committee concluded that embryo research was of substantial benefit. It recommended that embryo research should be permitted up to 14 days after fertilization, when the first signs of embryonic differentiation and organ growth occur and when implantation is largely completed. Fourteen days, incidentally, is also when a woman might perceive that she is pregnant as that is the time when she would miss her period. Another point which influenced the Warnock Committee's time limit was the fact that, up till 14 days, the embryo could not be regarded as a unique individual as twinning was possible until then. The Committee made a number of recommendations – in particular that a government licensing authority be set up to regulate matters relating to IVF, donor insemination, fertility treatments and embryo research.

The government was slow to react. Although debates on the report followed in both Houses of Parliament (and many MPs were concerned about embryo research), no government bill was introduced. The government felt it had more pressing business. A powerful lobby, lead mainly by the two organizations Life and The Society for the Protection of the Unborn Child, called for a ban on embryo research. They sought a Member of Parliament who would take up the issue, and were fortunate when that great champion of causes, Mr Enoch Powell, won the Private Member's Ballot to introduce a bill at the end of 1984.

Mr Powell's Unborn Children (Protection) Bill received its second reading on 15 February 1985. In his opening speech on that day, Mr Powell emphasized his feeling of "revulsion and repugnance" at the destruction of embryos "for the purpose of the acquisition of knowledge". Some listeners found it odd that Mr Powell did not appear to sense the same "revulsion" at embryos being destroyed (daily, in their thousands) by that popular method of contraception the IUD(coil). Was it then the "acquisition of knowledge" that caused Mr Powell so much personal distress? The ensuing debate was extremely revealing. Most MPs opposed to embryo research displayed remarkable ignorance about what was involved. In spite of numerous invitations from researchers, very few of them, including Mr Powell, had bothered to actually visit a department where embryo research was being conducted.

Mr Powell's bill had many glaring deficiencies. It required, for example, that all women having IVF treatment would require prior permission in writing from the Secretary of State. This infringement of personal liberty, completely unparalleled with any other medical treatment, was accepted without question by his supporters in the House of Commons, who mustered an astonishing majority of 172 votes at the second reading. This was particularly remarkable as Mr Powell's bill aimed to ban all research on embryos, except *where researched embryos were to be transferred back to the womb*. The appalling consequences of this – that women might deliver children which had been made abnormal by research – were pointed out to him, but he remained intransigent on this issue, as on virtually every other.

241

Although Enoch Powell's bill failed to get a third reading, it is remarkable that there have already been three more attempts to revive it. The last attempt, as recently as February 1989, was an identically worded bill introduced in the House of Lords by the Duke of Norfolk. It seems that the Duke, who at least took the trouble to brief himself by visiting research units beforehand, was unmoved by the many glaring anomalies in Mr Powell's bill – many people believe he was under pressure from the Roman Catholic Church to introduce such legislation. Perhaps his heart was not fully in it because, when he realized that his opponents were to introduce numerous amendments at the committee stages, he withdrew his bill (April 1989).

Not all Parliamentary activity has been negative. An all-party Parliamentary group called PROGRESS was set up after Mr Powell's bill foundered. It has been very influential in helping politicians understand why embryo research is essential. Many organizations involved with health care or handicap have joined PROGRESS, which still has important work to do if reproductive research is to be protected. PROGRESS needs membership; should you be interested in supporting its activities, please write to the address on page 245.

Government legislation on reproductive technology

In November 1987, after an extended period of consultation, the government produced a White Paper on reproductive technology. It proposed setting up a licensing authority to regulate all aspects of *in vitro* fertilization, and a free vote on the question of embryo research. However, so far, although the White Paper has been debated, no government bill has been forthcoming.

Doctors and scientists have been left to regulate themselves. In 1985, the Royal College of Obstetricians and Gynæcologists, together with the Medical Research Council, founded the Voluntary Licensing Authority (VLA). This was meant as an interim measure until government legislation was passed. In fact, the VLA continues to police IVF in the absence of statutory control, and does so very effectively. There has been no case of unethical or dangerous research, and all clinics have voluntarily submitted to inspection and have agreed to the VLA guidelines. None the less, there is no doubt that the profession as a whole hopes for proper, sensible government

RESEARCH: ETHICS AND POPULAR ATTITUDES

control because only this can settle public anxiety about what might be going on behind laboratory doors.

Issues involving human reproduction have always raised strong feelings. Nobody doubts the sincerity of those who believe that the human embryo is a person entitled to full protection. However, that clearly is a minority view: over the last three years in Britain, there have been three national opinion polls and one medical research study, all of which clearly indicate that the majority of the British people feel that embryo research is right, particularly if it is used to combat genetic disease. One can only hope that, when Parliament does finally vote on the issue, it recognizes that we live in a pluralistic society. In such a society, the individual families affected by these catastrophic diseases should be allowed to have the final say in whether or not their own fertilized eggs may be used to alleviate their suffering.

Suggested reading

The Tentative Pregnancy: Prenatal diagnosis and the future of motherhood by Barbara Katz Rothman, Pandora Press, 1988. This is a particularly sensitive account of the problems involved in antenatal genetic screening and the decision-making process.

Coping with a Miscarriage by Hank Pizer and Christine O'Brien Palinski, Jill Norman Ltd, London, 1980. This deals with the medical and emotional aspects of miscarriage; it contains much useful information, though some is now a little out of date.

The Gift of a Child by Robert Snowden, George Allen & Unwin, London, 1984. This is still the most useful book for couples contemplating the decisions involved in donor insemination.

Human Reproduction and In Vitro *Fertilization* by Henry Leese, Macmillan Education Ltd, London, 1988. This is a clear and detailed account written by one of the most respected and innovative scientists in the field. Excellent background for those who want readable, in-depth information on IVF.

The Experience of Infertility by Naomi Pfeffer and Anne Woolett. Virago Press, London 1983. Still my favourite book on the feelings that people, especially women, have about infertility. The authors show great concern and sensitivity. A feminist book which offers great comfort to people with intractable infertility. The medical information in it is not entirely accurate.

Coping with Childlessness by Diane and Peter Houghton, George Allen & Unwin, London, 1984. A fine book, describing the feelings and experience of infertility; admirably critical and very honest.

Infertility: A sympathetic approach by Robert Winston, Optima, London, 1986. I hesitate to recommend my own book, but I believe it to be an accurate and careful account of the feelings, causes and treatment of infertility.

Everything You Need to Know about Adoption by Maggie Jones, Sheldon Press, London, 1987. A useful account of all aspects of adoption, practical and business-like.

Useful Addresses

United Kingdom

British Pregnancy Advisory Service (BPAS)
Austy Manor
Wootton Wawen
Solihull, West Midlands B95 6BX
tel: 05642 3225

CHILD
367 Wandsworth Road
London SW8 2JJ
Tel: 01 740 6605.

Family Planning Association (FPA)
27/35 Mortimer Street
London W1N 7RJ
Tel: 01 636 7866.

National Association for the Childless (NAC)
318 Summer Lane
Birmingham B19 3RL
Tel: 021 359 4887.

PROGRESS
27 Mortimer Street
London WC1.

Women's Health and Reproductive Rights Information Centre
52 Featherstone Street
London EC1Y 8RT
Tel: 01 251 6332

Useful Addresses

Australia

Adelaide Women's Community Health Centre
64 Pennington Terrace
North Adelaide
South Australia 5006
Tel: 08267 5366

Brisbane Women's Health Centre
P.O. Box 248
Woolloogabba
Brisbane
QLD 4102
Tel: 393 1622

Elizabeth Women's Community Health Centre
Elizabeth Way
Elizabeth
South Australia 5112
Tel: 252 3711

Helath Sharing: Women's Health Information Service
Information Victoria Centre
318 Little Bourke Street
Melbourne 3000

Liverpool Women's Health Centre
P.O. Box 65
Liverpool
NSW 2170

Women's Health Information Resource Collective Inc.
P.O Box 187
653 Nicolson Street
Carlton North
Victoria 3054

INDEX